Aquarobics

Aquarobics
The Training Manual

GLENDA BAUM MSc, MCSP, SRP

Roehampton Physiotherapy Clinic, London, UK

with illustrations by

Jane Ancona

WB Saunders

London • Edinburgh • New York • Philadelphia • Sydney • Toronto

WB Saunders is an imprint of Harcourt Brace and Company Limited

Harcourt Brace and Company Limited 24–28 Oval Road
London NW1 7DX, UK

The Curtis Center
Independence Square West
Philadelphia, PA 19106-3399, USA

Harcourt Brace & Company
55 Horner Avenue
Toronto, Ontario M8Z 4X6, Canada

Harcourt Brace & Company, Australia
30–52 Smidmore Street
Marrickville, NSW 2204, Australia

Harcourt Brace & Company, Japan
Ichibancho Central Building, 22-1 Ichibancho
Chiyoda-ku, Tokyo 102, Japan

A catalogue record for this book is available from the British Library

ISBN 0–7020–2234–9

Typeset by J&L Composition Ltd, Filey, North Yorkshire

Printed and bound at The Bath Press, Avon, UK

This book is dedicated to
Leora, Micah and Benjamin,
and any future as yet unconceived
grandchildren

Contents

SECTION I   WHAT IS AQUAROBICS?

SECTION II SPECIFIC POPULATION GROUPS

SECTION III AQUAROBICS TO PROMOTE HEALTH AND FITNESS

SECTION IV THE EXERCISES

Preface

In this sophisticated, technological world, it is pleasing that something as simple and natural as standing in chest-high water and moving rhythmically to music, should be such a rapidly developing activity. Such interest in aquatic therapy is because it is effective, holistic and, most importantly, enjoyable. Its underlying purpose is to promote health and well-being and encourage independence and self-reliance on the part of the user. It is increasingly used by the professional because it achieves quick results, and fosters active participation through self-education, as the techniques learnt can often be continued unsupervised in a local swimming pool. Hence the patient is encouraged to be self-reliant and prophylactically orientated. The specific effectiveness of aquatic exercise arises from certain fundamental differences between exercising immersed and conventional exercise. Most importantly, performing the same exercise in and out of the water uses different muscles in different ways, as will be explained as the various themes in this book are developed.

Aquarobics is not really a new form of therapy, but more in the nature of new packaging on an ancient product. The difference nowadays, is that the underlying scientific rationale is known, and this helps to focus and increase the effectiveness of the therapy. The purpose of this book is to help professionals understand the underlying scientific theory, and thereby improve the practice. It is also to make available a basic vocabulary of exercises, with the knowledge of when, for whom, and in what circumstances they are appropriate.

But first, what do we mean by 'Aquarobics'? This word was coined, and first registered as a trade name in the UK in 1987, whilst the author was developing the concept of health-promoting or rehabilitative exercise-to-music-in-water classes. The word is not meant to refer simply to aerobics in water, but to a more general form of exercise incorporating multiple sections and aims. In 1987, a company called Aquarobics was formed by myself and a colleague to promote this new form of exercise and to train highly professional teachers of it. Since then this form of exercise has become popular, so popular that there is a danger of the word being used generically. It should, however, in the UK, only be used to describe Aquarobics classes taken by teachers who have been trained by Aquarobics Ltd or, latterly, Aquarobics Teacher Training. In order to use the name, teachers have to pass an examination, agree to adhere to a code of conduct that limits the number of clients in their classes and agree to continue their professional education by going on at least two days a year of upgrading courses. The majority of Aquarobics teachers are fitness coaches, physiotherapists, dancers or midwives (who are normally only certified to teach ante- and post-natal Aquarobics).

In this book, the word is used in a more generic sense. This is not intended in any way to weaken the legal position, which is that, in the UK, it should not be used to describe aquatic exercise, unless the professionals involved fulfil the above criteria.

Exercising in water is profoundly different in certain fundamental aspects; it is not simply a dry land movement that has been converted to the water. It is hoped that with a deeper understanding of the rationale behind water exercise, professional standards will rise and aquatic therapy, particularly using the holistic, Aquarobics philosophy, will become more widely available to the exercising public. The same basic principles apply regardless of whether the reason for exercising is for rehabilitation following injury or disease, for the prevention of degenerative changes, or simply to improve basic fitness levels. These are simply different aspects of the same continuum of 'movement-related-people-care'.

How To Use This Book

This book is being written on several different levels for at least three different groups of professionals. Firstly it is being written for physiotherapists, to give them the basic practical and physiological knowledge to be able to treat patients in the water better. It will assume an excellent knowledge of anatomy and physiology, and merely highlight the differences between aquatic and conventional exercise. However certain areas will be new — possibly the basic physics, some of the exercise physiology and particularly the section on the use of music. The chapters dealing with specific populations may highlight factors which are relevant to water, but which would not have been considered during normal physiotherapy.

The second 'client' group are physiotherapists who have already undertaken a postgraduate hydrotherapy course. They will probably only benefit from the sections on the use of music and the enhancement of general fitness and well-being (Section 3). This book should not present them with any conceptual difficulties, but should nonetheless be of value. The more you know, the easier it is to learn when encountering something new, but the more important is that little bit of new knowledge, and the associated widening of applicability.

Finally, this book is intended as a course book for professional dry-land exercise and fitness coaches who wish to convert their dry-land skills to the water. Such people will have a lot to learn, and for them it is hoped that this book will not only be a course text, but will continue to act as a 'user-friendly' reference manual. However, it must be stressed that whilst fitness coaches can become Aquarobics teachers for the healthy public, they in no sense become qualified as *therapists*. That requires the full rigour of a 3-year course of professional higher education.

If you would like to find out more about becoming an Aquarobics teacher, telephone 0181 876 7789.

Whichever career path has brought you to this book, it is hoped that it will be an easy, practical read and a future source of reference. However, teaching people movement skills in water is in itself a practical skill, and one which is made harder (but more effective and enjoyable) by the use of music. It is strongly recommended that you supplement this book by taking a short practical course to develop the particular teaching skills necessary in the acoustically hostile pool environment.

Glenda Baum

Acknowledgements

In this, my third book, I owe a great debt to my husband, Harold, who has been immensely supportive. He has acted as editor, proofreader, scientist-in-residence, and even computer-hack. He has tolerated mountains of paper and mess and weekends of solitude when I have been otherwise engaged. To him I pledge this to be my last technical book. Similarly, but not so intensively, I would like to thank the rest of my close family. From now on they will have most of my attention.

During the time this book has taken to write, I have organized the weddings of both my daughters, and have become a grandmother thrice (twice, I hasten to add, through the courtesy of my married son). Moreover, I have had two editors at Harcourt Brace who have produced three babies — Gill Robinson had one at the start and Miranda Bromage now has two sons. I hope the antenatal section was of use.

The physiotherapists and administrative team in my Practice have kept it running, and to them I am grateful. Especially so to Vicky Ware, Jane Featherstone-Witty, Carol Cass, Marcelle Foster and Caroline Alexander, who have read sections of the manuscript and given me valuable suggestions, and to Jacky Mandy and Angela Moran who kept the Practice ticking over.

Within the world of aquatic exercise, I would like to thank my Aquarobics partners Jenny Brown and Celia Carron, who have always been there to answer queries and provide useful opinions, Judy Jenkins and the National Organisation for Water Fitness for permission to use their safety material and for lots of other help.

Other professional colleagues who have helped are Gisela Creed, Sarah Mitchell, Sarah Murdoch, Yvonne Rogers, Alison Skinner and especially Jane Hall, who has been most helpful and supportive.

Finally, I am grateful to the many friends and colleagues from other countries: Igor Burdenko, Mary Essert, Susan Jackson, Jane Katz, Ruth Sova and Irene Wallin, to name but a few. I thank them for their friendship and the warmth of their welcomes, in this international club of aquatic enthusiasts.

Glossary

Aetiology (US Etiology)

The cause or causes of a particular disease.

Agonist / Antagonist

An agonist is a muscle acting on its own, or in combination with other muscles in such a way that its active contraction causes movement. The contraction of an agonist is associated with the relaxation of the muscle doing the reverse movement, known as the antagonist. For each movement at each joint, there is an agonist, the contraction of which necessitates the relaxation of the corresponding antagonist.

Atlanto-occipital joint

The joint between the head and the neck.

Atrophy

A wasting or shrinking of a tissue, e.g. a muscle, after it has developed completely and achieved its full size.

Coach

A trainer or teacher of exercise and health-related fitness. These terms are used interchangeably.

Cystic

A tissue which has developed pathological cavities.

DIP (Distal inter-phalangeal joint)

The joint nearest to the tips of the fingers and toes.

Haplotype

Genetic make-up.

Leukocyte

Any of several nucleated cells that occur in blood or tissue fluid, exclusive of erythrocytes and erythrocyte precursors. A kind of white blood cell.

MCP (Metacarpo-phalangeal joint)

The main 'knuckle' joints of the fingers.

Metastatic

Secondary growths of malignant tumours.

MTP (Metatarsal-phalangeal joint)

The joints between the toes and the rest of the foot. In the big toe, this is the 'ball' of the foot.

Neural tension signs

A clinical sign that indicates that a nerve, when stretched, is under undue tension.

Perineum

The tissues forming the base of the pelvic cavity, in front of the anus. In women, it is the skin, the vulva and the underlying sling of muscles.

Physical therapist

The name given to a physiotherapist in the USA.

PIP (Proximal inter-phalangeal joint)

The joint in a finger or toe which is nearest to the MCP or MTP (see above.). This excludes the thumb and big toes, which have only one such joint. Please refer to DIP above.

Polyarthritis

A type of arthritis that involves many joints.

SLR (Straight Leg Raise)

A test that is used to assess the presence of sciatica. The client lies supine, and one leg is raised as high as possible, with the knee in extension. It should go to about 85°.

Subluxation

A transient dislocation.

Teacher

A trainer or coach of exercise and health-related fitness. These terms are used interchangeably.

Thermoneutral

That temperature at which a resting, immersed body will neither lose nor gain heat. It is therefore at or just below normal body temperature.

Xiphisternum

The prominent process palpable at the lowest part of the sternum.

Section I
What is Aquarobics?

1

Exercise in Water

Land Versus Water Exercise

People of diverse capabilities can benefit from exercising in water because water is a totally different medium to air, and exercising in the former is physiologically very different from exercising in the latter. Many pages of this book will be used to clarify and explain the differences, but a key point is that people are virtually weightless when they are standing chest-high in water. Exercise on dry land can be dangerous, as manifested by the number of patients requiring medical or physiotherapeutic help after incurring sporting injuries. Such injuries occur either through heavy falls or because of the overloading of body tissues. Because the body is virtually weightless in water, not only are such injuries almost impossible, but people who are already injured, or in pain for other musculoskeletal reasons, are able to perform movements when immersed that would not be possible, or would be extremely painful, on dry land.

The Continuum

Such injured people might be elite athletes, exercising in water to maintain their aerobic fitness when prevented from exercising conventionally.

At the other end of the spectrum are severely disabled people who can only move without pain when immersed in water. Between these two extremes would typically be a 'normal' person who has recently recovered from a prolapsed disc. At what point are we talking about therapy, and when does it become therapeutic exercise to maintain health and increase fitness? This continuum of people is regularly encountered when dealing with exercise in water. Exercises led by a therapist in a hydrotherapy pool (or possibly even an appropriate swimming pool) are therapeutic in character by the very fact of being conducted by a therapist. They are 'medically orientated'. However, once the therapist has discharged the patient, the fitness professional may take over. Sometimes there may be a period of overlap when both work in cooperation for the greater benefit of the client. The two professions have different skills and knowledge bases, and all professionals should be aware of their personal limitations. As a general guideline, therapy should be carried out by the trained medical therapist, but this should not take away from the importance of the role of the fitness teacher in maintaining and improving the overall level of fitness thereafter.

The purpose of this book is to increase the knowledge base of both physical therapists and aquatic exercise coaches. It is not to turn the latter into the former.

Complex issues can always be reduced to the lowest common denominator and, in the case of aquatic exercise, there is the basic fact that a given volume of water weighs about 750 times more than the same volume of air. This difference in relative density between water and air is responsible for water being the kinder and more flexible medium in which to exercise. This will be explained in detail in Chapter 3.

Historical Perspective

Immersion has been used for therapy and relaxation for at least 2000 years. In Europe, spa therapy has been practised, periodically, since Roman times, and still is to this day. In the late 18th century, Society in England considered this a fashionable and beneficial activity, from the Prince Regent and his Court downwards. 'Taking the cure' was probably more effective than most other remedies offered by the doctors of the time – bleeding, purging, cupping, etc. – and it was certainly safer!

There are now well over a thousand active mineral and sea-water spas in Europe alone. The traditional philosophy at a spa was to 'take in' the waters – and this was done through every available natural orifice of the human body. It was, and still is, the custom to bathe in the waters, usually taking the form of sitting, floating or swimming. The exercise is normally gentle because the water is hot, and vigorous exercise could lead to hyperthermia. Moreover, floating is often easy, as many spa waters have a high salt content and therefore give great buoyancy. The anecdotal benefits of such spa therapy are many, and these are backed up by copious scientific studies, although many experiments were not very rigorous in their procedures. An indication of the perceived value is that many European health insurance systems willingly pay for rehabilitation treatment at spas.

Why Not Swim?

The concept that exercising in water is beneficial is not new, as for many years the medical professions have advocated swimming as the 'best' form of exercise for people with chronic musculoskeletal and other medical problems, because it is a non-weight-bearing activity. However, swimming, in common with almost all other forms of sport, has its inherent drawbacks. There are several swimming strokes, none of which take the major joints through their full range of movement. Moreover, a breast stroke kick is not good for knees, and is not advised after injury or malfunction to the knee joint. Necks are also at risk if breast stroke is not performed correctly, as a commonly performed way of swimming with this stroke is to keep the face out of the water. This puts an extension strain on the neck and can lead to pain in the neck, shoulders or arms. The biggest disadvantage of swimming, though, is that it does not capitalize on the physiological effects of hydrostatic pressure, as the whole body is too near the surface. This issue will be dealt with in detail in Chapter 3.

Hydrotherapy Training in the UK

In the UK, physiotherapists have practised hydrotherapy for many decades, and it used to be part of the basic training curriculum. Nowadays only about one-third of physiotherapy training courses include hydrotherapy, and the average time spent learning this speciality is 3 hours per student (Atkinson, 1996). There are, however, postgraduate courses available to familiarize therapists with the basic techniques of hydrotherapy, and specific methods such 'Bad Ragaz' and 'Hallewick'. Such methods are largely used for either one-to-one therapy, or group work for specific client groups, usually children.

The Availability of Pools

Traditionally, hydrotherapy for musculoskeletal problems has taken the form of gentle exercise carried out in small, purpose-built hydrotherapy pools. Such pools were kept at a temperature just a few degrees below normal body temperature, so the exercise had to be gentle. These pools are very expensive to build and maintain, and are therefore few in number. Perhaps if the pools were larger, as they are in other parts of the world (such as Australia and Japan) they would be more cost-effective. Because of financial pressures, many hydrotherapy pools, although small, are now 'hired' out to patient self-help groups when not required for hydrotherapy. This is welcomed by groups suffering with ankylosing spondylitis or rheumatoid arthritis, as people with such complaints are more comfortable in the tepid water of hydrotherapy pools than they are in the cooler water of swimming pools.

So What is Aquarobics?

Aquarobics is a system of exercises to music performed in water, which are health-promoting, natural, enjoyable and holistic. The majority of the exercises are carried out in the vertical position, in chest-high water. Movements are as functional as possible and are planned to involve the whole body, although in a therapeutic context there is more emphasis on any injured part. Exercises are structured in a logical way that is commensurate with current practice in the coaching of health-related fitness exercise (i.e. there is a warm-up and cool down). The various components of fitness (muscular strength and endurance, cardiovascular fitness, flexibility and general well-being — both physical and psychological) are considered and incorporated.

The Aquarobics system encompasses a wide range of activity, so that it can be used by professional physiotherapists and hydrotherapists as a technique for the rehabilitation of injured or disabled patients. Because, though, of the simple nature of the movements, it can also be used by fitness coaches in a swimming pool in order to get their clients 'fit', and keep them so, whatever their age or physical endowments. The word Aquarobics is a registered trade name in the UK, and can only be used to describe aquatic fitness classes, or their teachers, who have been trained and certified by Aquarobics Ltd and who abide by the Company's Code of Practice. This involves observing safety rules concerning the number of clients in sessions and the maintenance of professional teaching standards through attendance at courses for continuing professional development.

The Importance of Exercise

A certain amount of exercise is necessary to maintain good health (London Health Education Authority, 1994; Pate et al., 1995). In the western world, people now have an enormous array of exercises from which to choose. This is a comparatively recent phenomenon, as in former times in what is now the developed world, and today in large parts of the third world, exercise is not normally a recreational activity for the masses, but an essential part of normal living.

As with other things in life that are considered 'good for you', the benefit of exercise is only true up to a point. An excess of anything is harmful, and certainly an excess of exercise can damage one's health! This is either immediate damage at the time because of injury, or it could be a cumulative long-term degeneration caused by overuse. Possibly, the form of exercise is 'unnatural'. Skiing, for example, although invigorating, and enjoyable to many people does bear a high risk of damage, particularly to knee joints. Was it perhaps invented by an orthopaedic surgeon? The problem is that the basic design of the human frame is incompatible with the forces placed through the knee joint when falling whilst wearing skis, even with the most sophisticated of safety bindings. So what *are* we designed to do — what is natural?

According to Darwin's theory of evolution, every one of the millions of species of plants and animals that now live, or used to live, on this planet have had to adapt, through the selective process known as evolution, to a changing environment or risk becoming extinct. *Homo sapiens* is, biologically speaking, just another species. Our bodies have not really evolved since well before the stone age; indeed, there are a few people living today in remote parts of the world who still live stone age lives, and their bodies are fundamentally the same as ours. It could then be extrapolated that our human bodies evolved in order to lead the existence of early *Homo sapiens* — the hunter gatherer. Such a life would not have meant sitting for perhaps 50–60 hours a week on furniture, whether a hard office chair, or a soft sofa. Such a life would have involved short, sharp bursts of regular exercise: in order to gather food, it would have been necessary to

climb trees, hunt animals, grub for roots and mill and crush food, all 'by hand'. All of these activities are energetic, as are the survival strategies to escape from predators.

When at rest, a frequently adopted position would have been squatting. This was also essential for key aspects of personal hygiene as there were no seated latrines. It is likely that squatting was also a position of comfort, as can still be seen in certain parts of the world today.

Nowadays, most of the innermost workings of the body are known and understood. It appears that all parts of the body, whether one is looking at whole systems (e.g. the musculoskeletal 'macro' level), or at individual cells ('micro' level), each have a function to perform. Furthermore, it can be argued that if that function is not carried out, then malfunction is likely to result, and that this malfunction will then affect other systems. For example, if the musculoskeletal system is prevented from normal activity by, say, immobilizing a whole leg and foot in plaster of Paris for a few weeks, because of fracture to one section of it, then all the joints in the leg will be stiff when the plaster is removed. Also, the muscles which had been encapsulated will have wasted and be unable to contract as well as the muscles of the unaffected limb.

Every joint in the body has a range of movement which is normal for that joint. If it is not taken through this normal range, then problems will develop. In the same way that a car needs to have its engine started from time to time, our joints need to move to keep them lubricated.

Our bodies evolved to squat. When squatting, the hips and knees are in extreme flexion, but there is no strain on the joints if this has been practised since childhood. My own observations in travelling in parts of the world where squatting is still practised, are that osteoarthritis in the hip and knee joints is very rare, whereas in our society, the joints most affected by 'wear and tear' in ageing are those same joints, together with the spine.

Squatting is perhaps the 'natural' way to defecate and (in females) urinate. It is rarer to have weak pelvic floor muscles, and stress incontinence in cultures which do not use modern lavatories, as control of the pelvic muscles is learnt early in life, so as not to wet the feet! (It is true that in some such societies there is a high incidence of incontinence, but this is due to damage to the pelvic floor during protracted childbirth without medical intervention.) Other possible benefits of squatting include the reduced likelihood of developing haemorrhoids or varicose veins. Finally, observation made in the capacity of a physiotherapist treating patients with disc prolapses for over 35 years, shows that the agonizing pain that such patients feel when coughing or sneezing is reduced or much minimized if the same manoeuvre is performed whilst they are in the squat position. Therefore squatting must reduce intradural spinal pressure, and lack of regular squatting may even, therefore, be a factor in the development of the disc prolapse in the first place.

So having advocated the health-promoting advantages of being in the squatting position, you may wonder what its relevance is to aquatic exercise.

Squatting and Aquarobics

Squatting is considered a dangerous exercise on dry land. Most people cannot squat with their heels touching the ground because the unstretched tendo-Achilles get shorter. Whether or not the heel touches the ground, the squat position is 'provocative' to the menisci that are situated between the bone ends deep within the knee joint. In former decades, orthopaedic surgeons would request physiotherapists to do 'provocative' knee exercises in order to establish whether a meniscus was torn, and needful of surgery. Frequently, getting into an unexpected squat did actually cause the injury. It has therefore become accepted practice to discourage squatting, and this message has been disseminated through teachers of physical education, so that young children are also discouraged from squatting.

In recent years there has been a disturbing increase in the number of young people with chondromalacia patellae (pain at the front of the knee joint). This painful condition limits the ability to participate in sport and, if severe, may lead to degenerative changes in later life. Perhaps it occurs because children are designed to squat and they are now being discouraged from so doing? At any rate, it is far beyond the scope of this book to question such a basic dry-land exercise standard regarding the pros and cons of adopting a squatting posture. But any damage that is likely to occur will be because of the weight through the bone ends. Gatsi (1991) investigated the forces produced in the legs when squatting. He concluded that the femur and tibia have little contact, and the weight is primarily supported by the heels in the full squat position in subjects who were habitual squatters. Moreover, he believed that squatting cannot be responsible for osteoarthritis of the knee. When squatting in water shallow enough to prevent the face from getting wet, there is virtually no weight going through the knee joints, so it is no longer potentially hazardous, provided that Achilles tendons are still flexible enough to take the stretch.

Walking Correctly

Walking is an activity that we all do, but perhaps not in the most natural way. A small child walks using its entire foot, but in different positions at different stages of the gait cycle. First comes the 'heel strike' when just the heel is in contact with the ground, then as the weight goes forward onto the foot, the whole foot is in contact, apart from the arches, those intrinsic springy bridges that allow the weight of the body to be transported without damaging the tiny joints. Finally, there is a push from the big toe which transports the weight of the body forwards, but with a slight upwards cushioning. That is technically correct gait but, in our Western culture, where children are placed in shoes with rigid soles, and fashion dictates strange unnatural heels, gait pattern becomes sloppier. The way most people walk is rather like the feeling of holding two kippers by the tail, one in each hand, and flopping them down onto the floor. It is as though the majority of people have kippers at the end of their legs, instead of lively, active feet, consisting of many joints and muscles all working together in perfect harmony.

The footprints left in the sand by people who do not wear heavy clompety shoes is totally different from those that do. Correct, natural walking can be re-educated on dry land, but it is much easier to relearn in the weightless medium of water.

These two examples, squatting and walking, illustrate a basic philosophy of Aquarobics, musculoskeletal fitness can only be fully achieved by exercising in the way that our bodies were evolved to move.

The Aquarobics Population

Reference has already been made to the 'continuum' of people who can benefit from aquatic exercise, and it encompasses almost everybody. However, whereas the young fit person has the option of numerous dry-land alternatives, the water is a particularly suitable place to exercise for those aged over 60, those who already have fragile bones or joints, or those who are pregnant. The reason for this is that exercising in water is safer than dry land, because the forces put through joints are much reduced. Thus people can perform activities in water which would be painful, hazardous or just plain impossible out of the water. Moreover, because the muscle work is much more balanced than an equivalent dry-land 'work-out', it is particularly appropriate for people whose muscles are not so strong in the first place.

On the other hand, because of the high relative density of water, the young fit person can get a reasonable cardiovascular work-out — by working against its buoyancy and resistance — although they may not be able to engender sufficient forces to over-develop normal muscles (see Chapter 16).

Working with groups

Aquarobics can be done individually, as part of an individual hydrotherapy session or as one-to-one coaching in the fitness context. However, it also lends itself to a group activity — indeed there is a certain enjoyment which comes from being in a group and working (some of the time) in unison. This is a similar appeal to participating in a choir, formation dancing or possibly even team sport. A particular advantage of being in water is that the very nature of the medium allows for a flexibility of effort (e.g. same frequency of a movement, but different range) thereby making it a feasible group activity for people with diverse fitness levels. It is possible for all participants to stick to the rhythm, but varying the speed of the movement (because of the different range) dictates the effort. This will be dealt with in Chapter 5.

Enjoyment

If there is a secret ingredient in the succesful Aquarobics recipe, then this surely is it. A sense of the ridiculous is an asset, and a sense of fun is an essential. Ideally, all those in the water should be wearing a smile. It is, after all, quite ridiculous to be standing in chest-high water swinging a leg, or jumping about like somebody half your age. All of this done to enjoyable music — possibly even with a little communal singing thrown in. For myself, having the ability to make people laugh, and hence give pleasure, is a wonderful way to earn a living. Aquarobics instructors are not necessarily comedians and laughter is not an essential part of Aquarobics, but enjoyment is — and both are excellent forms of therapy especially for those whose lives are normally blighted with pain and misery.

Immersion and Exercise – The Component Features

There are two components to exercising in water: firstly the fact that the body is exercising, and secondly that this is happening with most of the body immersed in water. Both of these components have positive effects on basic physiology and it is hoped that the beneficial results of the two components taken simultaneously is greater than the sum of the two taken separately. How this might be the case will become clearer as the various features of aquatic therapy are considered in detail in the rest of the book.

References

Atkinson K (1996) *Undergraduate Training in Hydrotherapy – HACP Survey, Preliminary Results.* Aqualines: Hydrotherapy Association of Chartered Physiotherapists, pp. 7–9. (Available from the Chartered Society of Physiotherapy.)

Gatsi L (1991) Biomechanical measurement during squatting. *Proceedings of World Confederation for Physical Therapy.* Book 3, p. 1301.

London Health Education Authority (1994) *Moving On.* International perspectives on promoting physical activity. Consensus on the message for promoting physical activity in England and its delivery through a national strategy. 213. London Health Education Authority.

Pate RR, Pratt M, Blair SN *et al.* (1995) Physical activity and public health: a recommendation from the Centres for Disease Control and Prevention and the American College of Sports Medicine. *JAMA* **273**: 402–407.

2

Exercise Physiology

This chapter is a revision of basic exercise physiology. It is also hoped that it will fill the knowledge gap that exists for many professional therapists, who gain a detailed knowledge of physiology in the course of their training, but who are not necessarily familiar with current practice of exercise professionals in search of 'fitness' for their clients. It also aims to help Aquarobics coaches who are not necessarily sufficiently familiar with underlying physiological changes that happen when a person starts to exercise on dry land. It is necessary to understand some of the basic tenets of exercise physiology as they refer to conventional, non-aquatic exercise, in order to understand the differences when exercising in water. There is a suggested reading list at the end of this chapter for those who consider that their knowledge of conventional exercise physiology is too superficial. On the other hand, those with a good knowledge of both exercise physiology and current accepted practice within the exercise profession, may wish to move directly on to the next chapter, which will deal with the physiology of immersion.

The Concept of Fitness

When exercising in water, the response of the body differs in certain profound physiological respects from when doing the same exercises on dry land. The differences affect most of the physiological systems in the body, particularly the cardiovascular, the musculoskeletal and the excretory systems. These changes are beneficial, and therefore enhance the health promoting effects of moderate exercise. Most people participate in exercise because they want to 'feel fitter', and it is reassuring to know that this can be achieved in the medium of water, where the risk of injury is extremely rare. In other words, you can achieve the benefits without the hazards: the gain without the pain.

Although competitive sport, and associated skills training, can be traced back to ancient times, the idea of the general populace training to increase basic levels of fitness over and above the requirements of day-to-day living, is a recent phenomenon, and one which now has major commercial implications. When big business is behind exercise for health promotion, then the fitness of the nation takes on a new significance!

So what do we mean by fitness? Fitness is a multi-faceted concept, with different needs and levels for different people. The fitness needs of manual workers or athletes are greater than those of sedentary people. Are all sports people 'fit'? Is a professional rugby player who cannot easily bend down to tie his laces, 'fit'? Is a competitive weightlifter, who cannot jump over a low fence in order to catch a bus, 'fit'? Is a person with a chronic disease, such as asthma or ulcerative colitis, 'fit'? It could be argued that the rugby player and the weightlifter are not fit, because they lack flexibility and specific skill coordination respectively, but the 'sufferers' may be fit because, although, in one respect unhealthy (the World Health Organization definition of health is 'a state of complete physical, mental and social well-being, and not merely the absence of disease or infirmity'), their ability to perform a range of physical tasks may be over and above the requirements of their actual, normal daily activities. Does the question 'fit for what?' link needs to objective physiological outcomes of exercise? Can you be fit if confined to a wheelchair? What is the relationship between fitness and health?

There are many definitions of fitness; here is one more, that to some extent, addresses the above questions: 'Fitness is a state in which the body is able to undertake all normal activities, including moving quickly, yet have sufficient reserves to be able to cope with additional, unexpected, sustained but reasonable demands without undue exhaustion or injury.'

If asked for yet another definition, then most people would equate fitness with cardiovascular (CV) function. Certainly aerobic fitness is a common reason given for exercising and there is a known correlation between this and the prevention of coronary heart disease. The improved stamina that comes from aerobic training is important, but so are the other physical components: muscular strength and endurance, and flexibility. However, a person is not just a body, but a body and a mind encapsulated in a total system. Certain less-tangible aspects of fitness, such as feeling good and being mentally alert are as important as heart and musculoskeletal function. Exercise can enhance this psychological well-being as well as the physical aspects.

Perhaps the heart is the key to this holistic approach to fitness, because blood is the universal currency of all systems within the body. Every cell needs an adequate supply of blood to bring oxygen and nutrients, remove waste products and conduct chemical messengers which act as controls of the miraculously complex animal that is *Homo sapiens*. This can only happen if there is an efficient heart to pump blood round the enormous network of arteries, veins and their associated capillaries, and efficient lungs to load the red cells with oxygen and remove the carbon dioxide afterwards. This is, of course, a gross simplification, because the circulatory system itself is not just a passive system of tubes, but a dynamic network that must also function properly, as indeed must all other related systems (e.g. the kidneys). All of them are to some extent interdependent, especially when under stress such as exercise.

Similarly, the functioning of skeletal muscle cannot be considered independent of the heart. In order to exercise to improve muscular endurance and muscular strength, the peripheral working

Table 2.1
The components of fitness

Cardiovascular Heart and lungs and blood vessels
Muscular Strength and endurance
Flexibility Joints, muscles, connective and nerve tissue
Enhanced well-being A positive attitude to life without undue anxiety or depression

muscles need an adequate blood supply, and can only continue to contract if the heart is able to work at a sufficiently high intensity to pump the blood round the body to those same muscles. Even so-called 'anaerobic' muscle work is limited by the subsequent ability of the cardiovascular system to replace and recycle the organic molecules which fuelled the contraction.

The Effects of Exercise on the Components of Fitness

Cardiovascular Function and Exercise

There are about 5 litres of blood in the body, although its distribution between tissues varies with physiological state. All tissues, but especially the brain and nerves have a required minimum blood supply, and this is broadly equivalent to the amount they receive during sleep. The functioning of the CV system depends on demand, and the control mechanisms are extremely complicated and efficient. The body does not waste energy, and the heart only pumps to the level required. Blood supply gets directed (by the contraction or opening up of relevant circulatory pathways) to the active tissues on demand, e.g. to the gastrointestinal tract after eating to assist in digestion, to the skin if the core temperature rises, to assist thermoregulation, or to the working muscles when exercising.

Cardiac output (CO) is the amount of blood pumped around the body in one minute. It is the product of the heart rate (HR) — the number of beats per minute, and stroke volume (SV) — the volume of blood expelled with each beat. At rest in an average individual, at a heart rate of 70 beats per minute, and a stroke volume of 70 ml,

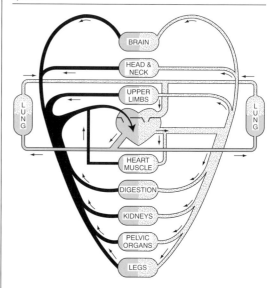

Figure 2.1 Schematic representation of the cardiovascular system.

about 5 litres is pumped through the left ventricle around the body per minute. At moderate exercise, at a heart rate of, say, 140 and a cardiac output of, say, 150 ml, 21 litres are expelled, which means that the entire blood supply is being pumped around the body about four times every minute.

Blood Shunting

When exercising at a moderate level on dry land, when the demand from the working muscles can exceed the supply, additional blood is made available by diminishing or shutting down the supply to non-essential tissues. Thus the metaphorical tap is turned off and the abdominal organs, the guts and the kidneys have their supply dramatically reduced. The blood supply to the kidneys is switched off by the antidiuretic hormone. This will be discussed in more detail in Chapter 3, as there are major differences in the pattern of blood-shunting when the exercise is in water.

Problems can arise from competing systems. After a meal, blood is directed to the splanchnic circulation of the guts. Heavy exercise at the same time then conflicts with demand for blood; hence the danger of vomiting or cramps when swimming in the sea immediately after eating.

Target Heart Rate

There is a linear relationship between oxygen consumption (demand) and heart rate (supply), almost to the point of maximum possible activity. The former would be a direct measure of any individual's aerobic efficiency (VO_2 max, or maximum rate of oxygen consumption). This direct maximum measurement requires the measuring and analysis of expired air and can therefore only be made under medical supervision with special facilities available.

The relationship between oxygen consumption and heart rate in any individual is a measure of the amount of oxygen delivered per heart beat, which in turn reflects the stroke volume as defined above. When looking at population data, rather than individual data, at differing work intensities, it has been established that the maximum possible heart rate and aerobic efficiency are age- and sex-related. This data has been converted to tables, so that one can read off and therefore estimate any one individual's maximum heart rate and aerobic efficiency, providing the heart rate is determined whilst doing exercise where a measurement of the amount of 'work' performed is also being made (e.g. using a bicycle ergometer at known speed and resistance). This 'work' measurement indicates oxygen consumption; it gives a figure which is the theoretical volume in litres of oxygen that is available to working muscles (including the heart muscle itself), per minute. By dividing by body weight, the data is adjusted so that different individuals can be compared.

Aerobic function tests should only be looked on as giving a broad indication of any one individual's aerobic capacity. It is probably accurate and useful to compare data collected in identical situations, but at different times (e.g. before and after a 6-week period of exercising), but it is not possible to infer from such a test how any individual would respond if actually asked to work to their maximum.

As therapists we know that in order to improve specific function (e.g. of an injured muscle) patients need to do repetitive, specific exercises, but we usually do not have the time or facilities to be able, in parallel, to work heart and lungs hard enough to bring about some improvement in cardiac function within the context of the regular specific therapy. However, in Aquarobics, such a desirable outcome of enhanced fitness becomes a practical possibility.

Training Effect

The human body is a highly integrated, extremely complex and energy-efficient machine. Like all good machines, if kept idle, it will eventually not function as well as it should; 'use it or lose it'. Muscles are meant to contract and joints are meant to move. If denied the exercise necessary to do this, then the muscles will get weaker, less bulky, more flaccid and waste away and the joints will get stiff. The heart, which is merely a very specialized muscle, also needs to be worked hard from time to time, or it too will function less efficiently.

So exercise is necessary in order for the body to function normally; the musculoskeletal and cardiovascular systems 'decline' if kept immobile. If those same systems are exercised progressively and moderately hard, then there are tangible increases in performance and efficiency as measured by muscle bulk and aerobic fitness (as defined by a spectrum of physiological parameters and metabolic markers). These outcomes are known as the **training effect**.

Overload Principle

The gains achieved by systematic progressive training require a certain intensity of effort, and this is known as the 'overload principle'. This term usually refers to the musculoskeletal system but the principle applies to all challenged systems. In order to achieve a specific fitness goal, then the relevant tissues need to be challenged. In other words, if the goal is to achieve muscular *strength*, then the exercise must overload the particular muscle that is the target. This is done by making the selected muscle work so that it has to move a load so great that it can only do this about 10 times. Perhaps that same muscle will cope with another such 'set' of exercises later in the session, but there should be a sensation of having worked that particular muscle hard if the strength is to improve. On the other hand, if muscular *endurance* is the goal for that particular muscle, this can only be achieved by overloading the muscle by selecting a lesser load, but continuing for many more repetitions, thereby working the muscle more aerobically.

Cardiorespiratory Endurance

The ultimate task of the entire cardiovascular system and lungs when exercising is to deliver sufficient oxygenated blood to working muscles (and to remove metabolites, particularly carbon dioxide). To improve this ability the exercise needs to meet the **overload principle** by being aerobically challenging. A sign that the CV system is being overloaded is breathlessness, but this need only

be to the extent where conversation is still possible. This is known as moderate breathlessness, and to produce it exercises must be selected which work many major muscle groups. The duration of exercise at this moderate degree of intensity will depend on the initial fitness level and on whether one is trying to improve or maintain aerobic fitness. The American College of Sports Medicine (ACSM) recommends 20–60 minutes of continuous aerobic activity for healthy adults.

The heart rate that should normally produce a moderate degree of breathlessness is known as the **target heart rate**, and this is from 60% to 90% of the maximum heart rate. This is equivalent to 50–85% of VO_2max or HR reserve (ACSM, 1995a). There are several ways in which it can be calculated. A commonly used method is the Karvonen formula:

1. Subtract standing resting heart rate (HR_{rest}) from maximal heart rate (HR_{max}) to obtain heart rate reserve.
2. Calculate 50% and 85% of the heart rate reserve.
3. Add each of these values to resting HR to obtain the target range, for example:

Target HR = $[(HR_{max} - HR_{rest}) \times 0.50$ and $0.85] + HR_{rest}$

Unfit individuals would exercise to the rate given using the factor of 60% but the higher level (90%) can be used for fitter individuals who are accustomed to aerobic training. It is obviously dangerous to select too high a level. In the water, the target heart rate must be lower, but this will be explained in the next section.

All the information above refers to normal, healthy people. People who have recovered from cardiovascular conditions, such as a myocardial infarct (heart attack), or who have an increased risk of developing cardiovascular problems for other reasons, are often advised to exercise by their doctors. Similarly, exercise is frequently prescribed for people with raised blood pressure. As beta blocker drugs are sometimes used for patients in these categories, it is important to note that one major effect of these drugs is to lower the heart rate which will subsequently not rise in the usual way in response to exercise. Target heart rates based on the normal population data are therefore not only useless, but could be dangerous as they would predict a figure far in excess of that individual's capacity.

Rating of Perceived Effort

In the water, unless aquatic cardiac monitoring equipment is available, **rating of perceived effort** (RPE) is the easiest method for exercisers to monitor work intensity. This self-assessed scale (see below), is designed to give a subjective indi-

Table 2.2
Revised Borg scale for ratings of perceived effort (RPE) (Noble *et al.*, 1983)

0	Nothing at all
0.5	Very, very weak
1	Very weak
2	Weak
3	Moderate
4	Somewhat strong
5	Strong
6	
7	Very strong
8	
9	
10	Very, very strong; maximal

cation of cardiac function. There is a linear relationship between HR, VO_2 and RPE so that this test has become a standard tool in fitness testing (Noble *et al.*, 1983; ACSM 1995b).

Muscular Strength and Endurance and the Effect of Exercise

Fox and Mathews (1985) stated that muscle bulk and strength are best increased by high load/low repetition exercises. In the gymnasium, weight strengthening normally involves slow, controlled movements with a near-maximum load. It is not as easy to work immersed using high load and low repetition exercises, as weights are not effective in the water. A similar effect can sometimes be achieved in the water by using long lever-arms. In practical terms, this means keeping the limbs straight by having knee and elbow extended. Increasing the speed of movement, thereby increasing the resistance will also increase the effort considerably and so help achieve the goals. Alternatively, buoyant equipment such as woggles or floats can be pushed down in the water, but this does alter the muscle work (see Chapter 3). Comparative studies of muscle work performed when immersed and non-immersed, using underwater electromyography by radiotelemetry, indicate considerably lower recruitment of fibres when immersed (Woledge and Baum, 1996). Whereas, clinically, a subjective improvement in muscle function is demonstrable after aquatic strengthening exercise, the lower recruitment demonstrated by the above studies does seem to question the validity of the overload principle. When dealing with the average person in later life one would not expect to have to achieve such high levels of muscle strength and power, so sufficient forces may be developed in the water to improve muscular strength and, particularly, power. Further research is required in this area.

Flexibility

In the water it is sometimes hard to get an effective stretch when there is no body weight to apply the stretching force. Pushing downwards against the pool side, or another person, assists in getting an effective calf stretch. Stretches to the hamstrings and sciatic nerve can be performed by putting one foot on the pool wall and gently trying to straighten the knee. Quadriceps stretches may be done in the usual way, providing the knee range of movement is sufficient to be able to catch hold of an ankle or foot. This position is probably harder for an older person to maintain out of the water because of their diminished ability to balance. Stretching positions that are effective in the water are shown below.

Another helpful stretching manoeuvre is to squat. In shallow water this can be done vertically, but if the water is too deep, then an alternative squat can be done by holding on to the side of the pool, with the feet against the pool wall.

Figure 2.3 Hamstring stretch.

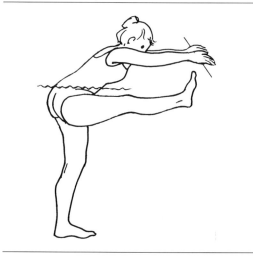

Figure 2.4 Quadriceps stretch.

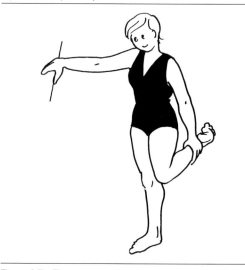

Figure 2.5 The squat.

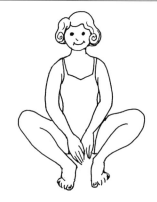

Figure 2.2 Calf stretch.

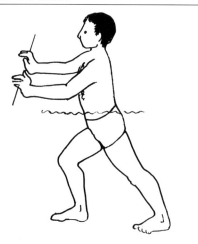

Table 2.3

Benefits of a moderate holistic long-term training programme

Lower resting heart rate and increase in stamina

Increased cardiac output and heart size

Increase in blood volume, number of red cells and amount of haemoglobin

Increase in muscle bulk, number and size of muscle fibres

Reduced body fat content (but not necessarily reduction in weight)

Improved flexibility

A sense of enhanced well-being and an overall improvement in functioning

Exercise for Rehabilitation – the 'Get-fit' Aspect

Having reviewed some technical, physiological aspects of exercise, let us return to the basic reasons for exercising; the attainment of the above benefits. In order to achieve them, it is implicit that the exercise required for any one individual must be at a fairly high intensity for that person. A certain degree of basic health is necessary in order to work enough muscles to put the cardio-vascular system into overload, and this is often not possible if one is dealing with 'patients' rather than 'clients' (see below). Earlier in this book, reference was made to the 'continuum' of people who might benefit from exercise in water. One end of this range is concerned with physiotherapy, and the object of the joint time spent by the therapist and the patient is to facilitate rehabilitation, promote the recovery of normal function, reduce pain, strengthen weak muscles or increase the mobility of stiff joints. This can happen either in a one-to-one situation, or within a group, or in a combination of the two where the therapist has a small number of patients, each of whom is performing their own individually prescribed exercises. In any of these instances, the subject will be referred to as The Patient, and the professional as The Therapist. This therapist could be a physio/physical therapist or a hydro-therapist, this latter term (in the UK) referring to an additional postgraduate qualification on top of the three or four years basic physiotherapy course. A shortened description of the objectives of treatment could perhaps be 'to get fit', as in all cases one is starting off with individuals with a specific impediment.

Exercise to Increase Fitness – the 'Super-fit' Aspect

At the other end of this continuum of people are those whose reason for exercising aquatically is 'to get fitter.' Such people might already be considered by others to be perfectly fit, and to be trying to become and remain 'superfit'. For example, it has become more common for professional or semiprofessional athletes to train aquatically once a week, to minimize the risk of injury caused by weight-bearing overuse, or trauma. In such a situation, the therapist concerned will be referred to as The Coach, and the subjects will be referred to as The Clients. The example selected refers to team training, and the coach, in this instance, could be the normal coach for the sport. It is hoped, however, that they will have undergone specialist aquatic training so as to make the best use of the water. In the rapidly expanding arena of exercise and fitness, the instructor may also be referred to as The Coach. S/he too will have undergone specialist, although much shorter, training. It is interesting to note that teaching and communication skills play a very large part in the jobs of both therapists and coaches.

Exercise to Maintain Fitness – The 'Keep-fit' Aspect

This group of aquatic exercisers is likely to be the largest, and perhaps one in which the range of fitness, abilities and expectations is the most varied. Within this group one would hope to find those people who have previously had physiotherapy for a musculoskeletal problem, such as low back pain, and been discharged from medical care with the instruction that they should continue to exercise aquatically to prevent relapse. One might also find sufferers of inflammatory joint diseases, such as rheumatoid arthritis or ankylosing spondylitis, who are in a non-acute state, who may well find exercising in water the best way to maximize their joint function, and who can work at improving overall fitness, including joint function, without the pain of weight-bearing activity. Other people in this group could be pregnant, elderly, overweight, or recovering from cardiovascular problems. They could, of course, simply be quite 'normal' individuals of any age or either sex, who elect to exercise aquatically.

Aquatic sessions for the specific patient groups mentioned above could be led by either a physical therapist, or a specially trained coach. There are not enough therapists, or warm pools, to be able to offer this service to all those who would benefit. That is not quite as sad as it seems, since there are psychological, motivational and cost-benefits if the patient groups fall within the 'exercise to promote health' arena rather than hospital-based therapy, and so attend exercise classes conducted by properly trained coaches rather than therapists. Specific chapters later in this book will relate to all those groups of people mentioned above.

Structure of a Session

To Begin – A Warm-up

Although very different in many important aspects, the exercise activity which probably bears the most resemblance to Aquarobics is a dry-land exercise-to-music class. This kind of class, as with virtually all schemes of supervised exercise, now follows a structure, and it is strongly recommended that a similar structure should apply to all forms of aquatic exercise. Any differences in structure arise because the risks of the two forms of exercise are very different. The risk of a participant in a dry-land exercise-to-music class getting hypothermia is extremely low, but the risk of a muscle injury is fairly high. In aquatic exercise, these two risk factors are reversed in importance.

In all exercise sessions there should be an initial warm-up period. The objective of this is to prepare the body for exercise, physically and motivationally. It should last 3–15 minutes, depending on the temperature and the individual circumstances. The movements should be large-scale and involve the major muscle groups and major joints, well within the comfortable range that is normal for each individual. This should raise the heart rate about 20–30 beats per minute, produce synovial fluid in the main joints and prepare the body for what is to follow.

The Middle Section – Know the Goals

Before starting any lesson, all teachers require some basic knowledge of their prospective students in order to calculate the aims and objectives of their class and produce (albeit theoretically) an outline session plan. The pre-session planning will involve obtaining the information necessary to make this plan. This applies equally to a physiotherapist, who may have already done a dry-land assessment, or a class Aquarobics coach who will have found out as much as possible about the fitness levels, needs and expectations required by his or her clients.

The aims and objectives of the above two scenarios are likely to be very different. Whereas the fitness coach will be planning a balanced total body fitness work-out, the therapist, who will probably have less time available, may have to confine him/herself to the affected part of the body. Nevertheless, it is often possible to work both the injured and non-injured parts so as to make the cardiovascular system work somewhat harder.

In a dry-land exercise-to-music class, an hour-long keep-fit class would, after warming up, probably first have an aerobic section lasting 15–30 minutes. This would consist of three stages: an easy initial stage in which the heart rate is gradually brought into the training zone, a long period, when this heart rate is maintained for most of the remaining time, and a final few minutes when the heart rate is allowed to drop to the pre-aerobic activity by slowing down and making smaller movements. The demand on the cardiovascular system at the peak stage is achieved by increasing the number and speed of working of muscle groups, and by raising the arms above the head. In an Aquarobics session,

this may be the only time that the arms are lifted out of the water.

In a therapy session, the exercises have a specific aim. This might be the improvement of gait, by walking in various ways, the strengthening of specific muscles or the gaining of a few more degrees of movement in a stiff joint. When doing gait re-training, the arms and trunk can be used to emphasize reciprocal movement. The hands pushing through the water, as in a military march, can be angled to increase the resistance and therefore increase the general workload. Experience has demonstrated that most people like to feel as though they are working hard, and enjoyment is conducive to effective therapy. If the aim is to increase joint range, e.g. to increase knee flexion, then walking with imaginary (or real, if the knee is strong and stable) flippers on the feet, with full reciprocal movement of the arms, takes attention away from the knee, and may sometimes gain the extra few desired degrees of movement.

In summary, a session needs a structure. It needs a beginning (a warm-up), a middle, which will vary, depending on the purpose of the session, and a cool-down. In water the latter must be short because of the risk of getting cold (see Chapter 3). In a health promoting class, flexibility is important, but muscle stretches are probably not essential. If they are going to be included, it is preferable to intersperse non-dynamic stretching exercises throughout the session, to prevent people from getting cold.

To Finish – A Cool Down

Accepted practice in the world of exercise is that a session should finish with a few minutes of exercising at a lower intensity, to allow the body to return gradually to its pre-exercise state. On dry land, it is usual to do some gentle stretching near the close of a session, particularly to stretch those muscles which have worked the hardest, and this may prevent post-exercise soreness. It is also common to take connective tissue to the limit of its range to encourage general flexibility. In the water, the decision on whether or not to stretch is not at all clear-cut. In the first place, in a therapy situation, stretching exercises aimed at specific stiff or injured parts, will probably already have happened. In any case it is usually impossible to stretch a muscle if the joints involved are restricted.

In the exercise class situation, rather than the therapeutic one, the only muscles which theoretically could get injured are gastrocnemius and soleus. This is because aquatic exercise often uses tip-toe walking, running on the spot or jumping, which are not done on dry land. There could, therefore, be overuse in the calves, if the heels are not placed down properly. Muscle injuries may have occurred in the water, but the only one that the author has come across professionally was a double adductor strain in a patient caused by attempting to carry out a star jump in the water. (The legs part and then come together in the space of one jump.) Because of the type of muscle work done (see Chapter 3), post-exercise muscle soreness is very rare, and therefore the need to stretch is for the positive reasons of increasing mobility, rather than the negative reason of preventing injury or soreness. More importantly, muscle-stretching involves minimal activity, and one cannot remain inactive in most pools without getting chilled. If, however, the pool temperature is above 31°C (90°F), then stretching and total relaxation whilst being supported in a floating position is, for many people, not only desirable but most enjoyable.

References

American College of Sports Medicine (ACSM) (1995a) *Guidelines for Exercise Testing and Prescription*, 5th edn, ch. 7. Williams & Wilkins, Baltimore.

American College of Sports Medicine (ACSM) (1995b) *Guidelines for Exercise Testing and Prescription*, 5th edn, p. 68. Williams & Wilkins, Baltimore.

Fox and Mathews, (1985) *The Physiological Basis of Physical Education and Athletics*, 3rd edn. Saunders.

Noble BJ, Borg GAV, Jacobs I, Ceci R and Kaiser P (1983) A category-ration perceived effort scale: relationship to blood, muscle lactates and heart rate. *Med Sci Sports Exerc* 15: 523–528.

Woledge R and Baum G (1996) EMG Study of Comparative Thigh Muscle Activity Dry and Immersed. Unpublished data.

Further Reading

Fox EL (ed.) (1989) *The Physiological Basis of Physical Education and Athletics*, 4th edn. Holt Saunders, Japan.

Bloomfield DJ, Fricker PA and Fitch KD (1992) *Science and Medicine in Sport*, 2nd edn. Blackwell Science, London.

3

The Properties of Water and Physiological Adaptations

In many ways teaching exercise in water is a lot harder than teaching dry-land exercise, whether the exercise is for rehabilitation (get-fit) or health promotion (keep-fit). There are many more factors to consider, such as the effects of the water temperature, the specific muscle work, the buoyancy of the participants, how one can overload, the risk of drowning, coping with difficult acoustics, summoning help if necessary, etc. Aquatic sessions must always be conducted by appropriately trained professionals. It is important to recognize that the professional hydrotherapist and the aquatically trained fitness coach occupy two different roles, which are often complementary to one another. Both sets of professionals need specialist training, and it is hoped that this book will assist in this. However, it must be stressed again that aquatic coaches are not qualified to provide rehabilitative therapy.

With that caveat we now come to a topic that both therapists and coaches need fully to understand if they are to become professional in conducting appropriate classes in water – the theoretical foundations underlying aquatic exercise. Those that think such exercise is just a soft option are mistaken. Aquatic exercise is, arguably, the most powerful modality of treatment available to the therapist and the safest medium in

which to exercise effectively so as to maintain and improve fitness. Below are the reasons why.

Hydrostatic Pressure

This is a force which applies to all surfaces of the body that are immersed in water. It is a function of water being relatively much heavier than air. The force increases with the depth of the water, and is multidirectional. It is the same force that affects divers, necessitating the need for decompression after deep dives. In a swimming pool this force is not dangerous, but beneficial. It could be said to be an inward 'squashing' force felt on the body.

Cardiovascular changes when immersed

Data obtained during studies of normal subjects sitting, at rest, immersed in thermoneutral water to the level of the xiphisternum, demonstrated a redistribution of blood and other fluids towards the centre of the body of about 700 ml, a resultant 34% increase in cardiac output, and a 700% increase in diuresis (Hall et al., 1990). These effects arise from the physical properties of water, specifically the hydrostatic pressure exerted on deeply immersed limbs. Hence such effects will be much reduced if the immersion is shallow, as when carrying out normal swimming.

It has already been stated that cardiac output is dependent on demand. As the above data was performed at rest, the increased cardiac output of 34% does not come from any demand from working muscles, but merely from the effects of the immersion, causing a redistribution of fluid. There is a resultant decrease in heart rate of about 10 beats a minute.

Although many comparative studies have now been carried out on cardiovascular function during conventional and immersion exercise, there is no consensus on the precise cardiovascular changes. This is largely because of the technical difficulties in equating the workload in and out of the water, because of the differences in the way in which muscles work (see below). However, it is accepted that exercise to a moderate intensity in warm water will result in a heart rate of between 10 and 25 beats a minute less than when working to the same *perceived* effort on dry land. This fact is particularly important when dealing with clients with cardiovascular problems.

The temperature of the water can affect the heart rate. Cold water can cause vasoconstriction in the legs, unless the intensity of the exercise generates enough internal body heat to counteract this. Vasoconstriction can theoretically affect blood pressure and possibly even heart rate, because of the shifts of fluid analogous to those referred to above.

Effects of Immersion on Respiration

There are changes in respiratory function both as a direct result of hydrostatic pressure on the chest wall and because of the central redistribution of 700 ml of blood. Overall, these hydrostatic and haemodynamic changes increase the work of breathing by 65% (Tipton and Golden, 1996). Vital capacity of the lungs is reduced by about 6%, but the expiratory reserve volume (i.e. the air retained in the lung at full expiration) is reduced by about 66%. Although these changes are not insignificant, there is no evidence that respiration is challenged in fit individuals. It must be remembered, though, that those people whose respiratory system is already compromised may find the additional pressure of water on the chest wall difficult to cope with. They may feel breathless, even when standing still. Immersion is therefore potentially hazardous to those people who already have reduced vital capacity or breathing difficulties, and may be considered a contraindication for aquatic therapy, although not necessarily an absolute one.

Effects of Immersion on the Excretory System

The study referred to above by Hall *et al.* (1990) shows a 700% increase in diuresis, the technical term for the process of urine production by the kidneys. In other words, when exercising in the water, not only do the kidneys fail to shut down to enable their blood supply to be diverted to working muscles, but their blood supply probably increases. Moreover, the kidneys themselves decrease their rate of absorption of filtered water (because of inhibition of the secretion of antidiuretic hormone) and produce seven-fold more urine than they would do in the same period, if at rest out of the water. This explains why most adults have a strong urge to urinate when they get out of the water, and perhaps also the urinary contamination of swimming pool water, usually blamed on children. Apart from the practical consideration that appropriate cloakroom facilities should be situated close to the pool, this may not at first sight seem relevant to exercise.

However, this loss of interstitial fluid from peripheral tissues, some of which is then excreted by the kidneys is a useful side-effect of exercise when immersed. It is the 700 ml re-distributed centrally because of hydrostatic pressure that inhibits the secretion of antidiuretic hormone. During energetic dry-land exercise, this hormone is secreted by the suprarenal glands and controlled by the pituitary gland. Related hormone secretions are responsible for the shutting down of the blood flow to the kidneys during normal dry-land exercise. The combined effect of these responses is a dramatic reduction in diuresis. This does not happen if the exercise is taken whilst immersed, and there are a number of conditions where this increased diuresis is beneficial.

Beneficial Effects of Immersion

Swollen joints are a common result of injury or other dysfunction. This is more frequently observed around the joints at the lower part of the body, the ankles and knees. This 'pooling' of fluid in the ankles and knees probably happens because of gravity and because of the greater 'uphill' distance from the ankles to the heart, as compared with the distance from the wrists to the heart. When immersed, regardless of whether this fluid is present because of musculoskeletal dysfunction, cardiac insufficiency (heart failure), or some other cause, hydrostatic pressure and the pumping action of leg muscles assist in its central redistribution. This is arguably the single most important reason for the effectiveness of aquatic exercise for the reduction of swelling

(and the resultant reduction in joint pressure and relief of pain) in the treatment of lower leg conditions. If this is so, then it should be pointed out that the same effects would happen equally well in a hydrotherapy pool or a swimming pool, providing that the exercise is performed in the vertical position, and the water is of equivalent depth. Theoretically, the deeper the immersion (chest-high rather than waist high), the more the reduction of swelling.

It has been observed that there is a reduction in lymphoedema in the limbs following aquatic exercise, but the beneficial effect is fairly transitory. In the arm, such lymphoedema can be the result of a radical mastectomy, in which lymph nodes and vessels have been removed. This compromises the peripheral lymph circulation. Although the benefit of exercise when immersed is short-lived, it is psychologically advantageous and may eventually be of more lasting benefit. It is not possible to immerse the arms as deeply as the legs, so the benefit will therefore be proportionately less than for legs. It must be remembered, though, that women who have had a recent mastectomy may be unable to go into the pool, as immersion may be a contraindication with radiotherapy. Moreover, the scar must be properly healed. Chemotherapy may also be incompatible with aquatic therapy because it may be too tiring.

Theoretically, Aquarobics for people with a mild degree of heart failure should be effective in the reduction of interstitial fluid by assisting heart and circulatory function and excreting some of this fluid (Warren and Come, 1988). It is more 'natural' to go to a pool and walk in water, than to take diuretics. There is an urgent need for further studies in this area.

In summary, hydrostatic pressure is responsible for the enhanced cardiovascular and renal benefits of aquatic exercise as compared to dry-land exercise. It can help to reduce swelling from injured limbs, and the resultant reduction in joint pressure is analgesic and conducive to further rehabilitation. It also perhaps explains some of the positive changes in feelings of well-being that have been reported by participants. There is an urgent need for research into all these aspects.

Turbulence and Resistance

The resistance encountered when moving through water is considerably greater than when performing the same movement in air, because of the increased relative density of the water. The degree of resistance offered by still water is dependent on the speed of the movement, and the shape of the moving part, and this happens because the moving part causes turbulence, i.e. random currents of water. To some extent, turbulence is visible. If one looks at the water in a swimming pool, which has been unoccupied and allowed to settle, it is possible to see a small object on the bottom — assuming of course that the quality of the water is sufficiently high not to obscure the vision. This is non-turbulent water. There will be minor currents, caused by convection as heat is lost from the surface, but generally the water is still. If there are people exercising or swimming in the water, it will not be possible to see the bottom, because the water will be in a state of motion.

Turbulence Used to Make Exercise Easier and Harder

We are familiar with the concept of streamlining — planes and boats are designed to be a 'pointed shape' so as to assist their passage through the air or water. Migrating birds are instinctively aware of streamlining, as they adopt a V-shaped formation to minimize turbulence. By so doing, the leading bird has the hardest task of 'breaking through' the resistance, and the other birds are, to some extent, drawn along in the slipstream. (Incidentally, the bodies of migrating birds are perfectly adapted to a streamlined shape, with their beaks pointing forward to 'cut through' the air.)

Moving through air or water sets up eddy currents which pull forward anything within them. There is a dead space immediately behind, and at an angle to the side (the same angle as the bird's adopt in the V-shape), and this means that there is much less effort for the person in the secondary, or subsequent positions.

An equally impressive effect is demonstrated by, say, a therapist walking backwards whilst creating turbulence with the hands; a patient walking forwards will then be 'drawn' with very minimal effort. This might permit a semi-paralysed person to get the feeling of walking forward, with only minimal muscle work. Generally, the less the turbulence, the easier it is to move against it. The slower the movement, the less the turbulence.

Important factors which relate directly to the degree of turbulence caused during any exercise are the speed of the movement and the length and shape of the moving lever. In circular movements, such as when a group of people holding hands move clockwise in a circle, this turbulence forms circular currents in the same direction, and the movement gets easier and easier because the eddy currents are set up in an orderly fashion. If, though, the group changes direction to move anti-clockwise, then they are having to fight against a wall of turbulence that is now in opposition, and much more effort is required.

In summary, the resistance caused by turbulence can make it easier or harder to exercise. Turbulence is minimized by moving slowly and by streamlining, and it is increased by quick movements and by selecting non-streamlined postures and equipment. On the other hand, the eddy currents behind a centre of turbulence actually facilitate movement.

Thermoregulation

The important topic of maintaining normal body temperature when immersed has been included at this point, because turbulence is the property of water that is most responsible for hypothermia. It will be remembered that heat energy is lost by the processes of conduction, convection or radiation. So how do these relate to 'Aquarobics', and where does the turbulence come in?

Heat is lost from the body much faster in water (a denser medium) than when exercising elsewhere, even though the ambient temperature in a gym or studio is likely to be much less than the water temperature. Turbulence speeds up the process of heat loss by increasing the amount of water that is in contact with the body (which, at blood temperature, is much warmer than the water in a normal swimming pool). This heat is lost to the water primarily by the process of conduction. Convection currents would form in still water, which would assist in the dispersal of heat, but turbulent water will speed up the process.

In all other forms of extended moderate exercise, the heat produced by muscle activity (normally an unwanted byproduct) will increase the core body temperature. In a swimming pool, though, the rate of heat loss by the above processes is so much greater than the gain, that the client is likely to cool down. This cooling can be coun-

teracted, to some extent, by increasing the overall rate of muscular activity, and planning the exercises so that there are bursts of activity interspersed with short periods of less activity.

Thin people lose heat more quickly because they do not have such a good layer of subcutaneous fat. (Fat is a good insulator, think of aquatic mammals.) On the other hand, obese people have too much insulation, and could theoretically be at risk from overheating. If such people are working aerobically in a hydrotherapy pool, which is frequently kept at almost body temperature, only a little heat will be conducted from their bodies to the water because of the small temperature differential. At the same time, their layer of subcutaneous fat will further reduce the conduction from their warm interior, and their core temperature could rise to hazardous levels.

Buoyancy and its Effects when Exercising

Everybody will be familiar with the story of how Archimedes, whilst bathing, suddenly understood why he was floating, and leapt from his bath shouting 'Eureka!'. What he had realized was that water imposes an upward force – buoyancy – on any body that is immersed in it. The force depends on the volume of water displaced. The weight of an object is a downward force. When a body is weighed in water, its weight is diminished by the upward force of the water's buoyancy. As Archimedes realized, when a body is weighed in air and then in water, the decrease in weight is equal to the weight of the water displaced by the object.

Obviously, if a body is less dense than water – i.e., a given volume of it weighs less than the same volume of water – its weight will decrease to zero before it is fully submerged. In other words, such a body floats once it has displaced a volume of water whose weight corresponds to the body's weight. Another obvious conclusion is that when pushing a floating object deeper into water an upward force will be experienced corresponding to the weight of the additional water now being displaced. In the case of a body of the same density as water, the net effect of its total immersion is that the downward force due to it own weight is precisely neutralized by the upward force of the water's buoyancy. In other words, such a body submerged in water behaves as though it is totally weightless, and its movement is only thereafter subject to other forces, such as turbulence.

But a person exercising while standing in water is not fully submerged, but is likely to be immersed to a level between their waist and shoulders. What percentage of weight (as measured on dry land) would be going through their feet? Harrison and Bulstrode (1987) found that this varied between individuals. The precise weight through the feet is dependent on body composition, particularly factors such as fat content (this will be explained below.) There are differences with age and gender, but Figure 3.1 demonstrates the approximate average values for percentage weight-bearing of the 18 subjects.

The principles that apply to flotation in water apply to any other medium in which a body is immersed. The denser the medium, the more buoyant it is. This consideration specifically applies when the medium is water in which significant amounts of salt are dissolved. Sea water is denser than fresh water, and hence more buoyant. Water saturated with salts, as in the Dead Sea, is so much denser than the human body that an average person becomes weightless, i.e. floats, when only very partially submerged, which is a very strange feeling indeed.

Figure 3.1 Approximate average values for percentage weight-bearing of 18 subjects. Xiph, xiphisternum; ASIS, anterior superior iliac spine.

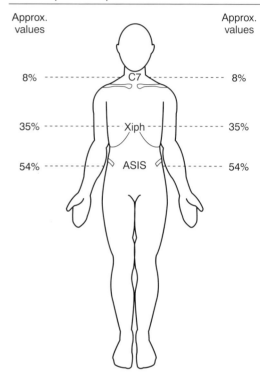

Approx. values

Approx. values

8% - - - - - - - - - - C7 - - - - - - - - - - 8%

35% - - - - - - - Xiph - - - - - - - 35%

54% - - - - - ASIS - - - - - 54%

There are three aspects to buoyancy which affect aquatic exercise. The first of these concerns whether or not people can float, the second relates to the use of equipment and the third, and most important, is that buoyancy has a profound affect on muscle activity in the water.

Who Can Float?

The human body is 55–75% water, which is why the relative density of an individual is not very different from water. Whether or not they can float will depend on two factors: firstly, the amount of air in the lungs and, secondly, their body fat content. The first factor is to some extent controllable, as it will depend on whether the lungs are inflated or deflated, but any additional buoyancy gained is only transient, until the air is expired. The second factor is permanent for that individual, unless they change anthropometrically, i.e. alter the ratio of their lean body mass to their fat content. Adipose (or fat) tissue is significantly less dense than water, bone, muscle or blood. This is why the cream floats to the top of the milk, and the fat to the top of the gravy. Overweight people have an excessively high fat content. On dry land this causes potential problems because this weight is an additional load on bones, joint and muscles. However, when immersed the relative density is much less, because this extra load is fat, and the person not only finds it easy to float, but may have problems re-orientating to the vertical position from the horizontal. On the other hand, athletic or lean individuals may find it impossible to float, because a higher ratio of their bodies is composed of muscle tissue, which is heavier than other tissues.

In studies in which large numbers of people have had their body density calculated, it becomes apparent that there are small differences between the 'norms' of different ethnic origins. For example, people of black African descent tend to have a higher relative density. They would therefore find it harder to float and to swim on the surface. This probably explains why black athletes often dominate the track and field events in athletics but do not tend to win gold medals at swimming.

Each individual has a centre of buoyancy, which is close to, but not in the same spot, as their centre of gravity. As body fat is usually concentrated around the abdomen, and as the lungs are central, then the centre of buoyancy is usually slightly in front of the centre of gravity, and slightly higher up the body.

Figure 3.2 demonstrates the centres of gravity and buoyancy in a 'normal' individual. It must be

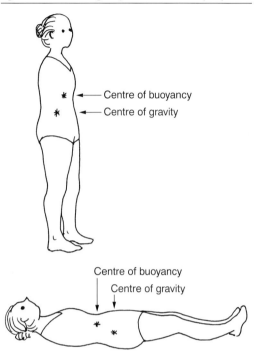

Figure 3.2   Centre of gravity and centre of buoyancy.

Centre of buoyancy
Centre of gravity

Centre of buoyancy
Centre of gravity

remembered that the arms may have a high fat content. In this case they will tend to float up to the surface. Lifting them up from the anatomical position would therefore require no muscular effort, but holding them down by the sides would require the shoulder adductors to work.

What Happens to Muscle Work in the Water?

The ability to identify which individual muscle or group is the prime mover in a specific movement is a basic skill of physiotherapy. To determine this, it is necessary to know which joints are moving, what the direction of the movement is, and how gravity interacts with that movement.

The work of maintaining an upright posture against gravity is primarily undertaken by extensor muscles, much more than their antagonists. Any movement that is performed in an upward direction, like going up stairs, is carried out with the extensor muscles working concentrically, whereas going down whilst also using the extensors, now uses them working eccentrically to control the downward movement lest it become a downward fall. In other words, the extensor muscle groups are more used than their antagonists. They are used both concentrically and eccentrically, and because of this dominant use, extensor muscles tend to have a preponderance of slow, Type II, aerobic fibres.

Figure 3.3 shows elbow flexion happening in two different starting positions. In both, the person is standing (not in water) in the anatomical position, but in Fig. 3.3(b), the left arm is horizontally abducted. The top row illustrates the exercise known in the fitness world as a biceps curl: the elbow is flexing as the forearm is lifted against gravity. The lower line illustrates a triceps curl, and the effort then goes not into the flexion, which is gravity assisted, but into extending the

elbow. A biceps curl works only the biceps muscle; concentrically going up, and eccentrically going down. The triceps curl works the triceps muscle, concentrically going up and eccentrically going down.

Now let us examine the situation when standing in shoulder-high water (Fig. 3.4). As already explained above, the downward force of gravity is more or less neutralized by the upward force of buoyancy. If one again looks at the exercises known as biceps and triceps curls, but imagines doing them immersed (Fig. 3.4) then the elbow flexion in (a) is produced by a concentric contraction of the biceps (exactly the same as when on dry land, but the return movement to straighten the arm is 'active' elbow extension, and is produced by a concentric contraction of the triceps. Similarly, if we examine the triceps curl (b), with the arm starting off floating, or immersed in the water, we can see that the buoyancy has counteracted the gravity, and the elbow is therefore flexed by the elbow flexors (the biceps) working concentrically. The reverse move-

---

Figure 3.3   Muscle work of elbow flexion and extension on dry land.   (a) Biceps curl   (b) Triceps curl.

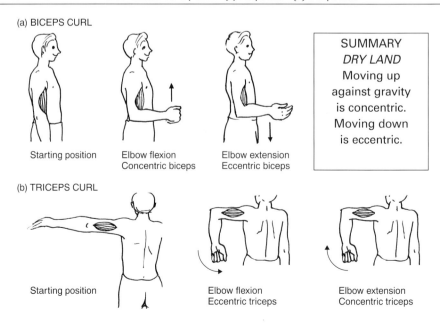

(a) BICEPS CURL

Starting position   Elbow flexion
Concentric biceps   Elbow extension
Eccentric biceps

SUMMARY
DRY LAND
Moving up against gravity is concentric. Moving down is eccentric.

(b) TRICEPS CURL

Starting position   Elbow flexion
Eccentric triceps   Elbow extension
Concentric triceps

ment, from the flexed to the extended position is produced by the elbow extensors (the triceps) working concentrically. In other words, the muscle work for both flexion and extension for both the biceps curl and the triceps curl is now concentric, as indeed it is for all movements in the water (unless buoyant objects are used, see below).

In other words, when immersed, both of these exercises would be better described as 'biceps/triceps curls', as the muscle work for both is the same, namely concentric biceps when flexing and concentric triceps when extending.

Muscle work using Buoyant Objects

Buoyant equipment is often used in therapy and aquatic fitness, either as support to maintain the supine position, or as an additional resistance in the same way as weights are used out of the water. The 'lighter' the object in relation to its volume, the more buoyant it is. However, whereas using weights on dry land does not alter the muscle work, but simply makes the same muscles work harder in the same way, using buoyant equipment when immersed totally alters the muscle work.

When buoyant objects are held in the hand, the real effect of the buoyancy is only felt if they are moved in a vertical plane. Any movement that takes place in a horizontal plane will not affect the muscle work, apart from perhaps working additional muscles in order to keep the float down. The muscles actually performing movements in a vertical plane, though, are the antagonists of the same exercise performed 'dry'.

Supposing we look again at the same two exercises used above (Fig. 3.5). In the first exercise, (Fig. 3.5a) the effort is in keeping the float under the water by keeping the arm extended. It is the air in the buoyant object that will bring it up and the triceps muscle which controls that upward movement. The triceps gets longer as the elbow

---

Figure 3.4 Muscle work of elbow flexion and extension with the arms immersed.
(a) Position of biceps curl exercise   (b) Position of triceps curl exercise.

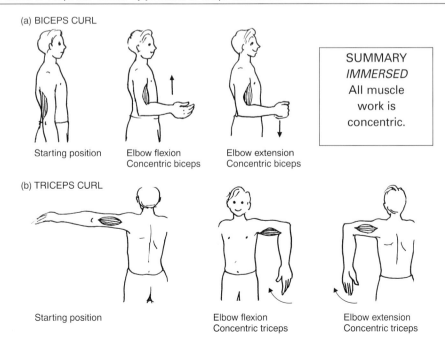

(a) BICEPS CURL

Starting position

Elbow flexion
Concentric biceps

Elbow extension
Concentric biceps

SUMMARY
IMMERSED
All muscle
work is
concentric.

(b) TRICEPS CURL

Starting position

Elbow flexion
Concentric triceps

Elbow extension
Concentric triceps

Figure 3.5   Muscle work of elbow flexion and extension when immersed and using floats.
(a) Triceps curl.   (b) Biceps curl.

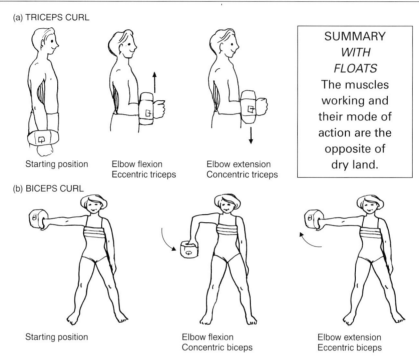

(a) TRICEPS CURL

Starting position   Elbow flexion   Elbow extension
Eccentric triceps   Concentric triceps

SUMMARY
WITH
FLOATS
The muscles
working and
their mode of
action are the
opposite of
dry land.

(b) BICEPS CURL

Starting position   Elbow flexion   Elbow extension
Concentric biceps   Eccentric biceps

flexes so this upward movement is controlled by eccentric muscle work of the triceps. Going down is a concentric contraction of the triceps. In other words, when holding a buoyant object whilst immersed, the exercise which, on dry land, is known as a biceps curl works only the triceps muscle — eccentrically going up and concentrically going down. Similarly the exercise which is known as a triceps curl in the gymnasium should be called a biceps pump when immersed and pumping down a buoyant object. Flexing the elbow is concentric biceps work and extending the elbow is eccentric biceps work.

To summarize:

1. All muscle work in the water is normally concentric.
2. When using buoyant objects in a vertical plane, the muscle work is the antagonist of

that on dry land, both in the muscle that is working and in the type of muscle work (i.e. concentric or eccentric).

Which Leg Muscles Work in the Water?

The elbow joint has been used to illustrate the above points, but physiotherapists are often more concerned with leg muscles than those in the arms. They may need to strengthen the quadriceps, hamstrings and gluteals as these have such key roles to play in normal ambulation and sport. All the variations of walking that can be done in the water use concentric muscle work, and one can certainly restore function and strengthen weak muscles when immersed because of the effort of pushing the water out of the way. Going forward has been said to work the anterior muscles and going backwards the posterior muscles, although no evidence has yet been published. However, an unpublished pilot study (Woledge and Baum, 1996) using underwater electromyography (EMG) did not confirm this. Further work needs to be done to clarify this.

Post-exercise Soreness

One outcome of the fact that all muscle work is concentric when immersed is that post-exercise muscle soreness is extremely unusual after a water work-out. Newham (1988) demonstrated that it is eccentric muscle work that can produce post-exercise pain, stiffness and fibre damage, whereas concentric exercise does so only rarely. Some people like to feel this soreness as they (mistakenly) feel it is the price to pay for the benefit of vigorous exercise. Such people need to be warned that this will not happen in the water — there are no muscular aches the next day, except possibly for patients with extremely weak muscles or some muscle pathology like fibromyalgia or wasting due to inactivity.

It should perhaps be reinforced that all the above applies only to the immersed situation: any muscle work that is done out of the water, such as having the arms reaching up above the head, or doing push-ups on the side of the pool, will be both concentric and eccentric and follow the usual 'dry' rules.

Summary

There are profound physiological differences between exercising conventionally and aquatically. The main reasons for this are the density of water, its hydrostatic pressure, turbulence, resistance, and buoyancy.

Hydrostatic pressure (i.e. the multidirectional pressure exerted by the weight of water) is depth-dependent and so, therefore, are the cardiovascular and renal effects. As these effects are beneficial, it is better to carry out most of the exercise when vertically immersed in water to about chest height.

The effect of turbulence and the increased resistance encountered when moving through turbulent water, can be modified to assist or resist exercise. The results are directly proportional to the speed of the movement and inversely proportional to the streamlining of the moving part. They are encountered in the direction of the movement.

Buoyancy is an upward force, and counteracts the downward force of gravity. Thus the body is almost weightless when standing shoulder-high in water, but the amount of weight actually going through the feet will depend on the ratio of fat to lean body mass in any one individual, and the degree of lung inflation.

Because of buoyancy, muscle work in the water is all concentric, and post-muscle soreness is very rare. The exception to this is when buoyant equipment is used. In which case the muscles working are the opposite group to those that would work on dry land: a biceps curl becomes a triceps curl and vice versa.

References

Hall J, Bisson D and O'Hare JP (1990) The physiology of immersion physiotherapy *Physiotherapy* 76(9): 517–521.

Harrison R and Bulstrode S (1987) Percentage weight-bearing during partial immersion in the hydrotherapy pool. *Physio Prac* 3: 60–63.

Newham DJ (1988) The consequences of eccentric contraction and their relationship to delayed onset muscle pain. *Eur J Appl Physiol* 57(3): 353–359.

Tipton MJ and Golden F (1996) Immersion in cold water. In: *Oxford Textbook of Sports Medicine* (eds Harries M *et al.*), pp 205–207. Oxford University Press.

Warren SE and Come PC (1988) Effects of water immersion in heart failure patients and in normal controls: Implications for volume regulation. *J Appl Cardiol* 3(3): 183–189.

4

Safety Considerations

Almost every activity in life has its potential hazards. Even such a supposedly beneficial, non-hazardous procedure, as rehabilitative physiotherapy, can sometimes rebound to result in the patient getting worse rather than better. Such a negative effect of therapy is less likely to happen during aquatic rehabilitation than with dry-land therapy. Similarly, all forms of aquatic exercise in swimming pools carry a lower risk of injury than, say, playing field sports. This is because the increased relative density of water makes it inherently a safer medium than dry land in which to exercise, and direct trauma which would result in injury on the pitch is extremely unlikely in water. The cushioning effect of buoyancy, turbulence and hydrostatic resistance, and the consequent dissipation of applied forces engendered, as well as the slower speed of movement in water are all reasons for the low incidence of injury. Moreover, high forces and pressures are less likely to build up within muscles, thereby reducing the risk of intrinsic muscle sprains and overuse syndromes. Finally, as already indicated in Chapter 2, buoyancy results in considerably reduced loads through joint surfaces, thereby dramatically reducing the risk of injury to bone surfaces or ligaments. On the other hand, aquatic exercise does carry the possibility, albeit extremely remote, of the ultimate hazard — death by drowning!

All of the above refers to the subject being in water. Unfortunately, the risk of injury to those professionals who are demonstrating exercises from the pool-side is probably greater than when teaching dry-land exercise. Not only are there the usual risks of falling, or of overuse muscular injuries, but the pool environment is inherently more dangerous than that of a gymnasium. The reasons for this will be elaborated later in this chapter, as will the other important aspects of injury: prevention and early management.

Before moving into the negative mind-set which is necessary for the 'what-if' approach of accident prevention, there are certain positive aspects of aquatic injury prevention which will now be considered. The first of these are the three Aquarobics principles.

The Aquarobics Principles

The following three principles have been developed to promote aquatic safety by minimizing the possibility of negative outcomes from aquatic exercise. It is strongly recommended that all Aquarobics participants (i.e. in both therapy and keep-fit scenarios) are familiar with them, at the beginning of each session.

(a) Do Not Push Through Pain

Aquatic keep-fit exercises should never be painful. Generally speaking, pain is a sign that something is not functioning correctly, and therefore has no place in 'normal' health promotion classes. Clients must therefore be warned that nothing should hurt, and that all stretches must be slow and gentle. There are occasions when it is desirable to move to the end of the normal range of movement of a joint, so that any further movement to that joint might cause a 'niggle' of pain, but clients must be made to understand that they have to cease the movement before the pain actually comes.

In hydrotherapy, on the other hand, it might be appropriate for the therapist to produce some pain, and this principle is more in the nature of an amber warning light than a red stop light. For example, the progressive mobilization of pathologically stiff joints is almost certain to be painful albeit less when the procedure is carried out in water. There will be other occasions that arise during therapy that are painful, but it is well within the remit of the physiotherapist to know when to 'push through the pain' and when not to, so as to advise the patient accordingly. As a general guideline, the patient should not feel pain if the therapy is taking the form of group Aquarobics, and should be told to tell the therapist if they feel any discomfort. It is then up to the therapist to decide whether or not to continue with that particular exercise.

(b) Movements Should Feel Good and Look Right

Newcomers to Aquarobics are more accustomed to being horizontal in a swimming pool than vertical. The usual balance and 'righting' reactions that keep the body over the feet on dry land, are not obvious in water. This is probably because the apparent reduction in body weight is not sufficient to stimulate the weight-bearing sensory receptors. As the underlying *raison d'être* of Aquarobics is to promote good health, this is achieved by performing the normal, functional movements and exercises which are required for life on dry land. There are, of course exceptions to this, as part of the joy of moving in water is to carry out unaccustomed movements and explore the new medium. However, generally speaking, if one wants to improve dry-land functional performance, then experience shows that it is better to exercise in the water in a way which is compatible with dry-land existence. Therefore, when performing a movement in the water, which could be done out of the water, it should be performed in such a way that on land it would not cause the client to fall over.

Similarly, the type and quality of movements selected should be aesthetically pleasing and feel 'natural' and 'normal'. Not only are such movements less likely to cause injury, but they should, theoretically, assist movement function when not immersed.

(c) Sensible Moderation

As already stated, injury or negative outcome are rare sequelae of aquatic exercise. The expected outcome is benefit. However, in the context of aquatic rehabilitation, when the desired outcome is an improvement, it is occasionally possible to get an adverse reaction. It could be said that the ability when immersed to use the musculoskeletal system to produce normal pain-free movements, when such movements out of the water would be painful or impossible, is a very powerful therapy. We are accustomed to other forms of therapy, such as pharmaceuticals, having adverse reactions, frequently associated with overdose. So it can be with aquatic therapy: a little too much of a good thing can be harmful.

Are There Any Dangerous Aquatic Exercises?

(a) In the Context of Hydrotherapy?

Theoretically, it is possible to envisage scenarios such as that of a patient being rehabilitated following an unstable spinal lesion, who could be told to do a particular movement, using too great a force, that might result in further damage. Assuming that the professional involved was in possession of all the clinical details, this damage could be said to be due to misplaced professional judgement, and is beyond the scope of this book. If, though, a therapist is conducting an active exercise session, then it is very unlikely that damage could be caused, providing the **Aquarobics principles** listed above are followed.

(b) In the Context of Aquatic Exercise?

Aquatic coaches will be aware that there are many exercises performed in non-aquatic classes that are considered contraindicated. These would include squatting, double straight leg raising, cycling with the spine supported on hands and the legs vertically in the air, and many others. Such exercises are dangerous because of additional loading through joints being put in compromising positions, or because the lever arm of movement is dangerously long, or because of misplaced momentum which is hazardous to joints. In the first two instances, the damage may happen because of the effect that gravity has in determining the mechanical nature of the acting forces. In the last example concerning momentum, it is the speed which is a vital factor determining the amount of force.

In all of these instances, the same exercise performed in the water would not be dangerous, assuming, of course, that it were possible to carry them out while immersed. The downward force of gravity is neutralized by the upwards force of buoyancy and, moreover, the forces are not only confined to the one joint, but dissipated to allow movement elsewhere. For example, if lying supine in the water, supported on floats, no strain is felt when both legs are lifted up. It is impossible to lift the legs more than a few inches, because the trunk gets deeper in the water to compensate as the legs are raised.

Exercises in which there is a surplus of momentum are very much harder in the water because the increased viscosity of water, as compared with air, means that the same speeds cannot be established.

An exception to the general principle that few exercises are contraindicated in water is when carrying out rapid, straight leg sideways kicking movements, e.g. a star jump, attempting to get the legs apart and together in the space of a single jump. It is possible for this exercise in water to cause actual injury to the adductor, and possibly even the abductor muscle groups in the legs, such as tearing the fibres, or pulling away from the bony origin. The forces involved are quite considerable, a combination of momentum and a very long lever. Moreover, this movement may have been performed in the past as a dry-land exercise without injury, and the memory of this can predispose to doing it over-enthusiastically, as the client tries to reproduce the former 'easy' movement without realizing the danger. This is the only aquatic exercise known by the author to carry a high risk of injury, and is therefore contraindicated except for extremely fit populations who have well-developed adductors, such as ballet dancers or hurdlers. Other exercises, if not performed correctly, can cause overuse injury; for example, if doing lots of running or jumping (both activities not necessarily normally performed), there can be problems in the calves if the heels are not placed down. Advice on lowering the heels is therefore an important teaching point.

Underwater EMG studies have shown that the level of electrical potential developed in working muscles, which is an indicator of the amount of fibre recruitment, is considerably and significantly less in the water than when performing an identical movement out of the water (Awbrey, 1996; Woledge and Baum, 1996). This is surely why it is very difficult to build up sufficient force in a muscle in water to actually injure the fibres.

Systemic Effects: The Importance of Observation

It is assumed that all professionals who are responsible for the safety of people undertaking exercise are familiar with the signs and symptoms of over-exertion. They may, however, not be aware of the signs of hyperthermia and hypothermia. The signs of all three conditions are given below.

Crisis Management

There are two aspects to risk assessment, and probably the most important of these is the

Table 4.1
Signs of over-exertion, hypothermia and hyperthermia

Body part	Symptoms/signs	Due to
1. *The early warning signs of over-exertion*		
Skin	Probable flushed, possible grey with white patches. The skin colour may depend on the water temperature — could be pale	Working at an unaccustomed intensity
Muscles	Muscle pain and cramp	Working at an unaccustomed intensity
Other organs	Can feel sick or vomit	Possible clinical predisposition, or heavy meal
Cerebral	Headache. Initially, not keeping up with the moves, becoming slightly uncoordinated	Possible clinical predisposition, e.g. high blood pressure
Respiratory system	Breathless. Unable to carry out a conversation. If activity level maintained, becoming distressed	Possible clinical predisposition, e.g. chest infection, asthma, etc.
Cardiovascular	Possible chest or arm pain, dizziness, collapse	Possible clinical predisposition, e.g. raised blood pressure, atherosclerosis, etc.

ACTION: Summon help (unless mild muscle symptoms only). If mild, keep them moving a little, and then get them out of the pool. If any cardiovascular signs present, get first-aider and dial 999. Stop class and prepare for cardiopulmonary resuscitation (CPR)

Table 4.1
Continued.

Body part	Symptoms/signs	Due to
2. *The signs of hypothermia*		
Skin	Very pale all over; if asked, will say they feel cold	A cold pool. People with low amount of subcutaneous fat, e.g. thin or old
Muscles	Shivering	Possibly those who have not been working at a high enough intensity
Cerebral	Becoming uncoordinated	A cold pool

ACTION: Escort out of the water immediately. Then first aid as appropriate: get dressed, blankets, warm drinks, etc.

Body part	Symptoms/signs	Due to
3. *The signs of hyperthermia*		
Skin	Very red all over, especially the face. Possible sweating in the part that is not in the water	A warm pool. Overweight and obese people
Muscles	Not performing as well	Possibly those who are unfit and unaccustomed to working at a high intensity
Cerebral	Possible headache, becoming uncoordinated	A warm pool

ACTION: Slow down the activity to minimal for a couple of minutes. Observe them closely. That should be enough to reduce the core temperature. If in doubt, have them get out of the pool and get dressed and rest somewhere with a cool drink.

prevention of accidents or other 'negative outcomes'. The Aquarobics principles above are one example of good practice designed to minimize the hazards. There are other potential hazards involving the pool, the pool water and the surrounding environment. No amount of planning can cover all eventualities as there is always a risk of something totally unexpected happening. There is therefore always a need for an emergency procedure, and this needs to be practised from time to time, so that all professionals near or at the pool-side know their roles.

Emergency Policy

Most industrial, civilized countries now have legal requirements and policies designed to prevent accidents happening. Initially such regulations applied mainly to factories but they now extend to all public places, including leisure facilities. In the UK, under this legislation, there must be a written Emergency Policy Action Plan that is specific to each unit within any organization. There are requirements that this policy will be known to all staff working in the area. To ensure that emergencies are properly reacted to, it is necessary to have regular practices, or simulations. In an aquatic environment it is essential that all personnel know the local emergency policy, and that new staff are familiarized with it as soon as possible.

All emergency policies applicable to water exercise facilities will assume the availability of certain rescue equipment, such as that necessary to assist in evacuation from the water. They will also require some kind of alarm system to summon help. Also, it is assumed that there will always be somebody present, close to where the exercise is taking place, who is fully proficient in cardio-pulmonary resuscitation.

The Prevention of Accidents to Clients

Major Risk Factors

Probably the three most important questions to be considered in the prevention of accidents to clients are the ability of the clients to swim, the presence of any contraindications or other medical abnormalities that would predispose to risk, and whether or not the session is being adequately observed. There are two aspects to this last point, firstly, are the number of participants compatible with safe observation and, secondly, does the person carrying out the observation have life-guarding skills?

CAN THE CLIENTS ALL SWIM?

The ability to swim is not a prerequisite for the participation in either Aquarobics or hydrotherapy. In fact, it may well be discouraged in the latter activity. However, most adults who cannot swim are nervous of the water, and should they slip there is more chance of a dangerous situation developing than would be the case for water-confident swimmers. Hydrotherapy pools are small, shallow, and have one or two staff members present. It is therefore extremely improbable that any potentially hazardous situation would happen because of the lack of 'water skill'. Such situations would be more likely to arise because of a medical emergency (see below).

Non-swimmers are at much greater risk in a swimming pool because of the slippery pool floor, and the lack of something to hold on to. There are other factors about the design of the pool, such as the angle of slope, which are a greater potential hazard to non-swimmers than to swimmers. Finally, the sheer size of the body of water means that if a non-swimmer gets into trouble, they may not receive the help they need, simply because nobody has noticed.

If non-swimmers are kept in the shallow end, and near the coach, and perhaps allocated to the observation of an appropriate other member of the class who is water competent – then the risk of hazardous situations developing is minimized. However, the legal responsibility for safety of class participants always rests with the person in charge of the session.

Another important factor in safety for the non-swimmer is to limit the number of participants in any session to an observable and manageable number, perhaps also restricting the number of non-swimmers.

ARE THERE ANY CONTRAINDICATIONS, SUCH AS MEDICAL ABNORMALITIES, THAT WOULD PREDISPOSE TO RISK?

There are a few definite contraindications to immersion, and several more factors which need to be taken into consideration, and may be contraindications in certain circumstances.

In the UK, the Hydrotherapy Association of Chartered Physiotherapists lists the following contraindications:

Table 4.2 shows conditions which are incompatible with hydrotherapy, in that the attached risks are too great, even for immersion within a hospital hydrotherapy pool where good medical back-up can be expected. The contraindication relating

Table 4.2

Absolute contraindications to hydrotherapy and aquatic exercise

People who are medically unstable, i.e. the relevant system must be stable, e.g. after a cerebrovascular accident (stroke) the cardiovascular system must be stable

Those in cardiac failure who are unable to lie flat without distress

Whilst the acute symptoms of a deep vein thrombosis are present

Angina or shortness of breath at rest

Status asthmaticus, i.e. a severe asthma attack

During a course of radiotherapy (if irradiated skin is to be immersed)

Acute, uncontrollable diarrhoea or vomiting

Proven chlorine sensitivity

Table 4.3

Probable contraindications for hydrotherapy; absolute contraindications for aquatic exercise

The presence of Venflon or Hickman's line *in situ,* or any other catheters

Low vital capacity

Hypotension or hypertension*

Epilepsy*

Vertigo

Unstable diabetes

Within 10 days of completing a course of radiotherapy

Systemic illness or pyrexia (fever)

Incontinence of faeces

Open infected wounds

Poorly controlled epilepsy

Known aneurysm

* Aquatic exercise may be possible depending on the degree of the problem and the amount of supervision.

to vomiting and diarrhoea is not so much for the protection of the ill person, but more as a public health measure to avoid pool contamination and hence the spread of infection.

Table 4.3 lists certain other conditions in which all the circumstances should be carefully considered before deciding whether or not the person may undergo hydrotherapy. Such people should, almost certainly, be excluded from aquatic exercise class, as the level of supervision and medical expertise there will be much less than for hydrotherapy.

There are certain dangers associated with specific population groups and these will be mentioned in greater detail in the relevant chapters which follow. However, for convenience the main points will be listed below, as it is appropriate here.

The Importance of Screening Clients

In a hospital setting it is likely that the medical and general status of any patient will be known, but their swimming ability is probably unknown. Good practice dictates that the patient will have a dry-land assessment before the immersion takes place. At that time patients can be asked to complete a screening form. An example of the one used in Roehampton Physiotherapy and Sports Injuries Clinic is given in the Appendix 4.1 to this chapter.

As regards health-promoting aquatic exercise, it is also considered good practice for coaches to carry out a written screening for potential hazards before a first participation. In the UK, this

Table 4.4
Special precautions necessary for aquatic exercise

Condition	Precaution
Mild hypotension or hypertension	Get signed approval from their GP, and have small class numbers and good observation
Asthma	Have inhaler at the pool-side, and adequate observation
Incontinence of urine	Adequate education, and a nearby toilet
Tinea pedis or verrucae	Some pools have specific policies. Perhaps wearing special rubber socks
Contact lenses	Should probably be removed
Hearing aids or grommets	Should not immerse above chest level. No swimming
Sensitivity to chlorine	It may be possible to have the chlorine at the lower end of the accepted level
	Careful showering afterwards
People with learning disabilities and those with mental health problems	Small groups taken by specially trained personnel or, if in a normal group, allocate a 'minder'

Table 4.5
Potential dangers with specific aquatic populations

Population	Hazard
Pregnant women	Joint injury if too vigorous
Older people	Hypothermia if thin and the water is below thermoneutral

is standard coaching practice as laid down in national coaching qualifications for sport and recreation (S/NVQ, 1997). It is important for the coach to have a written profile of potential hazards for all participants. Ideally this should be completed before the first attendance, so that the coach is aware of any limitations. In addition to this one-off detailed screening, the coach should carry out a brief verbal screening at the beginning of each session, to see whether any of the usual participants are injured or have other relevant problems. The written screening is harder to organize beside a swimming pool than in a gym because of the environment being wet, and the clients being cold and not having the necessary writing implements. Nonetheless it should be done, ideally before the clients get changed.

The UK National Organisation for Water Fitness (NOWFit) has adapted a screening form from the PAR Q pre-exercise questionnaire. This is intended for participants in aquatic fitness classes. This questionnaire, NOWFit's Code of Ethics and NOWFit's Aquatic Risk Profile all have safety implications. Copies of all these documents can be found in Appendices 2–4 of this chapter.

The Number of Participants

All group aquatic activities carry the remote but feasible risk of a person collapsing and remaining unnoticed in turbulent water. It is therefore essential that coaches observe their class at all times, only turning their back very briefly to demonstrate an exercise, for not more than a few seconds. Ideally there should be another person whose sole occupation is to observe the class and who is also a lifeguard. There should always be somebody present with the requisite lifeguard skills, but this may sometimes be the coach. Whereas this is perhaps acceptable in a shallow pool with not more than 25–30 participants, it is not enough observation in a large pool, or where there are a high number of participants. The Amateur Swimming Association (ASA) guidelines states that there should not be more than 30 participants in an aquatic class (ASA, 1996).

The National Organisation for Water Fitness recommends that class numbers do not exceed 30, preferably with a coach and a lifeguard. Although this is ideal, it is recognized that commercial considerations may make this impossible. When larger classes are taken and/or there is no separate lifeguard in attendance, the coach *must* be satisfied that, one way or another, all participants are under continuing observation, and that there is the means immediately to deal with any emergencies that might occur.

Prevention of Accidents to Professional Personnel

(a) In hydrotherapy

Whereas gentle hydrotherapy bears a low risk of hazard for both patient and immersed therapist, this risk rises if the therapist is directing the operation from outside the pool. This is because of the possibility of the therapist tripping over objects, or losing balance and falling into the pool, whilst absorbed in observing the patient rather than the pool-side surroundings. Such risks are comparatively low. There are, though, other small risks, which come from working in an environment where both the air and water temperature, and the level of chemicals used may be considerably higher than the normal non-aquatic working environment.

It is usual practice in most hydrotherapy pools for the physiotherapist to treat patients using handling techniques. This normally requires that they get into the pool with the patients but, whereas the patient may be in for 30 minutes to an hour, the physiotherapist may remain immersed for up to 3 hours. We have already seen that immersion causes marked physiological changes, and these would of course be happening to the therapist as well as to the patients. Indeed, because of the extended time that physiotherapists may spend immersed, it is surprising that negative effects are not reported more frequently. Hydrotherapists have been known to complain of tiredness and possibly a predisposition to catching colds or other minor ailments. There are also reports of allergic skin reactions, usually caused by the use of bromine as a disinfecting agent. Because of this, bromine is now seldom used, chlorine or ozone being the chemicals of choice.

(b) For the Aquarobics Coaches

The risk of injury is considerably multiplied in the case of an Aquarobics coach taking a fitness class from, what is known in professional jargon, as 'the deck' (in other words teaching from the pool-side). Moreover, participants must be restricted to water in which they can safely stand, and must be able to stand up from lying on their front and back. Such injuries can broadly be divided into two categories: first, direct trauma as the result of slipping and falling and, second, overuse injuries. Whereas most dry-land aerobics coaches teach on a wooden floor, which is 'sprung' to minimize impact, Aquarobics coaches who teach from the deck are standing on a ceramic tiled surface, probably rough or uneven (to render it supposedly non-slip). Moreover, any pool floor will be wet because of splashing. The hazard risk is increased because there is no ideal footwear. The teachers often opt not to wear trainer shoes (because of the difficulty of getting them on and off when going in and out of the water) and even if specialized impact-absorbing aquatic shoes are worn, the tiled surface will produce considerably more impact force through the coach's body than would a sprung wooden studio floor.

How then can one minimize the risk of injury to the coach? By having them teach, as much as possible, from within the pool. In fact, teaching whilst immersed has many advantages. Firstly, when performing any moderately fast exercise, it is impossible to move at the same speed in the water as it is when not immersed. This makes it very difficult to demonstrate certain activities, such as running or jumping – or, indeed, the majority of the exercises that are normally performed in an aquatic class! If one is trying to motivate the participants to move to the beat of the music, then it is harder from the deck, as it requires superior teaching and motor skills to demonstrate at (what feels to the inexperienced teacher) an abnormally slow pace. There are obviously occasions when it is necessary to demonstrate a lower body exercise, which would not be seen by the participants if the teacher were in the pool. In this instance, the coach would need to get out of the water to demonstrate.

Environmental Factors

Pool environments are considered by many to be hostile. They are wet, humid, hard, acoustically unfriendly and fraught with potential danger. One way to avoid dangers is to be aware of them.

Table 4.6
Issues of practical concern in and around a pool

1. The actual pool

Water quality	(a) Cleanliness – adequate filtration and disinfection systems. If water is at rest, a coin should be visible on the bottom
	(b) Temperature – appropriate for the activity: Hydrotherapy pool: 31–36°C, swimming pool 27–31°C
Pool flooring	Preferably non-slip. Watch out for cracks, drain holes, or differences in surface, e.g. shiny, slippery, stripes as lane markers
Water depth	Ideally, for aquatic exercise, about chest high. If deeper, how steep is the slope? Could a poor swimmer slide out of their depth?
Access	Is the access by ladder or steps? If the latter, are there handrails? Are the steps slippery? Would a disabled person be able to get in and out without assistance? Is there a hoist?
Rails	Is there a hand-rail to hold on to when exercising?

Table 4.6
Continued.

2. The pool and changing room surroundings

The surface	Is it dry or wet and slippery? Is it a deck level pool; if so, can you stand on the grid? Are there any loose or chipped tiles? Are there any grooves or uneven places? Is the surface (including grooves, dips, etc.) adequately clean and reasonably dry?
Toileting facilities	Are there sufficient, efficient toilets and showers? Is there access for disabled people? Are these areas adequately cleaned and maintained? Are there adequate facilities for hair-drying, make-up, etc.?
Seating for changing and resting	Are there enough hygienic seats so that elderly or balance-impaired people can sit down to get dressed? Is there some privacy for those that prefer it? Are there adequate secure lockers?
Overall access	Are there easy stairs with handrails and lifts?

3. Clothing

Clients	In a swimming pool, costume matters. Are they appropriately dressed? (Women's clothing should give breast support; either by wearing a bra or appropriate costume.) High leg costumes are revealing, shorts underneath provide modesty. Shoes are not necessary unless the water is below waist depth (when trainers with cushioned soles will reduce the impact)
Coaches	Their costume is even more important as, when demonstrating, it may have to cope with exercising in and out of the water. If demonstrating on the side, trainers should be worn. Coaches may need to watch their body temperature. Thin coaches could become hypothermic and may need to wear wetsuits to keep warm

4. Equipment

Floats, woggles, etc.	Correct procedures must be followed for lifting and storing equipment. These items are not heavy, but bulky and difficult to transport. All such equipment can get broken, especially items with straps. Care must be taken when instructing people how to use equipment. Poor swimmers could tip over and be in danger
Electronic equipment	All such equipment must be battery operated and not on mains electricity. Even where there is low-voltage mains available, flexes are a hazard, and somebody tripping could pull an entire music system into the pool, potentially electrocuting all pool occupants. Batteries are heavy, so care is required in lifting and handling
	One serious occupational hazard for aquatic coaches is the development of vocal cord polyps, because of shouting in the poor acoustic environment of a pool, possibly over the noise of music and swimmers. A battery-operated submersible head set (hands free) microphone is now available and very much recommended

This next section will examine aspects of the pool environment in respect of potential hazards. The total environment will be divided into four different areas: the actual pool, the surrounding and changing areas, clothing and equipment. For convenience, issues of practical concern that are not strictly hazardous are also included, as they will also normally be included in any environmental checklist.

There is always some risk of something going wrong, but assessing the likelihood of possible hazards and establishing procedures for dealing with them, cannot only minimize the damage caused, but could potentially save a life. It is also a duty of care and a legal liability. However, because accidents can happen, with no question of fault or blame, as professionals we have the inherent responsibility to ensure that our clients are protected as far as possible. It is not enough to be a really top-class professional, it is necessary to ensure that the unfortunate client, if injured, can get recompense and, in order to do this, there is a need for public and professional liability insurance cover. In an ideal world, this would be a statutory obligation.

References

Amateur Swimming Association (1996) *Safe Supervision for Teaching and Coaching Swimming.* Amateur Swimming Association.

Fuller RA, Dye KK, Cook NR and Awbrey BJ (1996) Electromyographic analysis of the quadriceps during partial single leg squats on land and at varied water depths. *J Ortho Sports PT.*

National Organisation for Water Fitness (1997) *Safety Guidelines for Aquatic Exercise.*

S/NVQ (1997) Revised Sport and Recreation Standards, Unit D43 for Coaching, Teaching and Instruction. HMSO, London.

Woledge R and Baum G (1996) EMG Study of Comparative Thigh Muscle Activity Dry and Immersed. Unpublished data.

Appendix 4.1   Sample form, Roehampton Clinic

ROEHAMPTON PHYSIOTHERAPY AND SPORTS INJURIES CLINIC
INFORMATION FOR POOL PATIENTS

We hope that you will enjoy the pool session and find it helpful.

Please note that the spa pool appears solid when it is not in use, as it has a white cover. Do not stand on it, or you will fall in and hurt yourself!

There are only two changing rooms, so these may need to be used by more than one person — but only one at any time. Please therefore put your clothes tidily and leave room for other people. There are plastic bags in the green string bags. These can be used for your underclothes, or to put your wet costume in afterwards. If you have any valuables, you may want to place them on the table outside, where they can be observed.

It is sensible to 'spend a penny' before entering the pool, and you may well find that you need to pay another visit when you come out. This shows that the hydrotherapy is good for the kidneys, and helps to reduce any swelling in your legs.

We try to keep the pool water as sterile as possible. Please always shower before and after entering the pool. The pool is used for people who have just had surgery.

It gets very slippery and can be dangerous — especially if you have crutches. Please move only slowly and carefully.

When you come out the pool, please help yourself to a clean towel. When you have finished with it, please put it in the basket.

When you are dressed, we ask you to sit down for at least 15 minutes in the Reception area, and have a drink which will replace some of the fluid you have lost. If you would rather lie down, then ask the Receptionist and, if at all possible, this will be arranged. It is normal to feel nicely tired after a pool session, and this is more marked if you also go into the spa.

PLEASE COMPLETE OUR RISK ASSESSMENT FORM.

RISK ASSESSMENT FORM

It is necessary to ask you some questions, to help us minimize any possible risk.

Please tick either the 'NO' or the 'YES' box, as appropriate.

Do you suffer from any of the following?

	NO	YES
FEAR OF THE WATER?		
CAN YOU SWIM?		
A HEART CONDITION OR HIGH BLOOD PRESSURE?		
DIZZINESS?		
BREATHING DIFFICULTIES?		
ASTHMA?		
DIABETES?		
SKIN ABRASIONS?		
ATHLETES FOOT OR VERRUCAE?		
ARE YOU PREGNANT, OR HAVE YOU HAD A BABY WITHIN FIVE MONTHS?		
ARE YOU ACCUSTOMED TO TAKING EXERCISE?		

ANYTHING ELSE WHICH MAY BE RELEVANT?

PRINT NAME ....

SIGNATURE .... DATE ....

CHECKED BY ....

Appendix 4.2   The British Universities and Colleges Physical Education Association (BUPCPEA) Risk Assessment Profile for exercise in general that has been modified to make it appropriate for aquatic exercise, by the National Organisation for Water Fitness (NOWFit).

BUCPEA / NOWFit RISK ASSESSMENT

NB Yes = Safe / Correct   No = Hazard

	Hazard rate	No	Yes	Action taken in response or comment
1.0 General				
1.1 Are exercises under the control of a qualified instructor from a recognised organisation?	4			
1.2 Is there a system to ensure that participants who have suffered medical conditions such as heart trouble, high blood pressure, back pain, asthma or are pregnant consult with the instructor before commencing exercise? Has a screening process been carried out to ascertain non / weak swimmers?	4			
1.3 In the exception of more than 30 participants in a class: a. Additional Lifeguards and / or assistant teachers should be present to maintain the ratio b. Does team teaching apply?	3			
1.4 Are all beginners given instruction before commencing exercise? Beginners should be briefed on: a. Maintenance and recovery of balance b. Posture and body alignment	3			
1.5 Are all users given warm-up and cool-down exercises as part of the programme?	3			
1.6 On deck, do instructors wear appropriate footwear such as trainers to cushion impact?	4			
1.7 Is the music at an appropriate volume to permit the instructor to be clearly heard?	3			
1.8 Has the pool bottom, shape and shelving been assessed in relation to lesson content?	5			

	Hazard rate	No	Yes	Action taken in response or comment
1.9 Is the pool surround free from obstacles, i.e. buoyancy/training aids when they are not in use?	5			
1.10 Are there regular checks by a named person on all equipment used?	5			
2.0 Classes				
2.1 Are participants: a. Individually assessed as to their ability before starting the course/lesson?	3			
b. Working at an appropriately paced intensity to suit their needs?	3			
c. Taught to recognise the onset of fatigue?	3			
2.2 Are the exercises adapted to the water depth?	5			
2.3 Are participants observed carefully to check that they do not over-exert themselves either physically or mentally and that the correct body position is maintained?	4			
3.0 Equipment				
3.1 Is the equipment inspected regularly?				

27.11.96

Appendix 4.3   Water Fitness Screening Questionnaire, National Organisation for Water Fitness (NOWFit).

Name: ....   Date of Birth: ....

Address: ....   Tel. No: ....

....   Doctor's Name and Tel. No:

....

1. Has your doctor ever said you have heart trouble?. . . . .   Yes/No
2. Do you ever have pains in your chest and heart? . . . .   Yes/No
3. Do you ever feel faint or have spells of severe dizziness?. . . . .   Yes/No
4. Has your doctor ever said your blood pressure was too high? . . . .   Yes/No
5. Has your doctor ever told you that you have a bone or joint problem such as arthritis that has been aggravated by exercise, or might be made worse with exercise?. . . . .   Yes/No
6. Is there any good physical reason not mentioned here why you should not follow an activity programme even if you wanted to?. . . . .   Yes/No
7. Do you suffer from diabetes?. . . . .   Yes/No
8. Have you suffered from epilepsy?. . . . .   Yes/No
9. Are you over age 55 and not accustomed to vigorous exercise?. . . . .   Yes/No
10. Are you on any form of medication?. . . . .   Yes/No
11. If yes, please state condition and medication. . . . .
    . . . .   Yes/No
12. Are you pregnant or recently had a baby?. . . . .   Yes/No
13. Do you suffer from asthma? . . . .   Yes/No
14. Have you recently had an operation?. . . . .   Yes/No
15. Do you have a hip/knee replacement? . . . .   Yes/No
16. Do you swim competently?. . . . .   Yes/No
17. What other exercise do you do. . . . .
    . . . .

If you answer yes to one or more of questions 1–15 you should consult your GP before participating in exercise.

I hereby acknowledge that the nature of the exercise class I am about to undertake has been fully explained. Whilst I am aware that all care will be taken, I do so at my own risk.

Signed: .... Date: ....

Appendix 4.4   NOWFit Code of Practice for Exercise to Music in Water

Swimming pool environment

1.1	Water quality	Systems are in place to ensure the following:
		Chemical levels are regularly checked and recorded
		Clarity of the water is of a high standard
		Temperature of water is checked and consideration given to class content as a result
		Basic pool environment hygiene standards are high
1.2	Written procedures	Systems are in place to ensure a SAFE working environment
		Emergency Action Plan — procedures to be followed during an emergency
		Normal operating procedures — potential hazards, first aid supplies, lifeguard duties, emergency poolside aids, health and safety issues

Safety Considerations

2.1 Classes should be limited to 30 participants per instructor

2.2 All participants should be screened via an appropriate questionnaire such as a PAR Q and this to be followed up by regular verbal screening and observation

2.3 Additional lifeguard cover should be present on pool side

2.4 Where lifeguard cover is not possible instructors should hold a basic life saving qualification, i.e. Rescue Test (RLSS), Bronze Medallion or NPLGQ

2.5 All instructors should hold a current CPR certificate

2.6 Unless specifically designed for pool side, all electrical equipment should be battery operated

2.7 Instructors should be familiar with the emergency procedures specific to the pools where they teach (Ref. 1.2)

2.8 Do instructors have their own insurance cover?

The Instructor

3.1   All instructors should be trained to meet the NVQ occupational standards for teaching non-swimming water exercise (Aqua) through an accredited organisation

3.2   An instructor should not teach a specialised area, i.e. deep water, 50+, ante/post natal, unless they have been accredited with recognised specialist training

3.3   Instructors should be responsible for assuring that their own working environment is safe, i.e.

> Not teaching on mats or trampettes

> Wearing well-supported footwear

> Ensuring that buoyancy/training aids are safely stored on pool side while teaching

3.4   Instructors should wear appropriate clothing with limited jewellery, i.e. no necklaces or dangly earrings

3.5   Instructors should not turn their backs on a class except momentarily

3.6   Instructors can enter the water provided it is *safe to do so*

3.7   Instructors are expected to update their training on an annual basis

3.8   Instructors should take care not to dehydrate and to encourage participants to drink sufficient fluid

5

The Use of Music

Moving rhythmically to music is not only one of life's great pleasures for most people, but is probably an instinctive pattern of behaviour. Nowadays, primitive tribal dancing to insistent, repetitive drum beats is found deep in West Africa or New Guinea and perhaps in inner-city discos. It is probable that such activity releases endorphins, which induce a feeling of euphoria and relieve pain. Exercising to music is therefore easier and may be more beneficial than without. Certainly, if the tape runs out during a session, and the music stops – the class loses its sparkle.

The Importance of Music

Aquarobics uses music for two reasons. First, it is enjoyable to move in water to music, and the pleasure is enhanced if more than one person is involved. The other reason is more technical. Assuming the music has a regular beat, and that movements are done in time to this beat, then the music indirectly dictates the amount of effort that is put into that specific exercise. However, as is apparent in any disco, it is possible to vary, according to individual choice and ability, the extent, and hence the speed, of movement that is in time with a particular beat. Very little effort is

needed to move slowly through water, but the faster the movement, the harder the work. This is because of the additional resistance of the water that is created by turbulence, which is one of the reasons why water is such a wonderful medium in which to exercise. It allows each individual to put in only the requisite amount of effort, and it means that people with very different fitness needs can appear to be doing the same exercise to the same music although they are, in fact, working at very different 'effort' levels.

Working to the Phrase and Beat

Those Aquarobics teachers who are also dry-land exercise-to-music teachers, will find that music has to be used in a different way in water. First, by far the majority of exercises have to be done much slower than on dry land. The additional resistance of the water makes it virtually impossible to do large-scale movements at the same speed. In fact, this is the great skill in being an aquatic teacher because, unless the teacher is immersed, they are likely to demonstrate the exercises much too quickly from the pool-side, and their clients cannot keep up with them. This is the commonest basic teaching error, and the result is potential anarchy. The clients work at their own speed — which has probably got very little to do with the beat of the music. In water, it is simply not possible to work to every beat of normal music. Regular exercise music is about 100–120 beats per minute, and the resistance of the water prevents moving that quickly. It is perfectly possible, and desirable, to work to every second beat (half-time), to every fourth beat (quarter-time), or to every bar, or even to a complete phrase.

The exercises selected should use these other tempi hidden within the regular beat, and tune in to the feeling that the music gives. If the piece selected is romantic and smooth, then the exercise should be flowing. If the music is Country and Western, then the movement needs to pick up the strong beat, and perhaps be slightly jerky and 'horse-like'. If a Souza march is being played, then march-like movements will feel appropriate. There is much more scope for creative choreography than in dry-land exercising.

It is difficult to talk about the choice of music, as this is such a personal issue. It is important not to dislike the music, but it is probably more important that it is enjoyed by the clients than by yourself. Choice of music is age-biased. A reason frequently given for ceasing dry-land exercise classes is the mindless music that is played.

In earlier generations, one had to make one's own music or find a rare live performance. Now that music is so much a part of everybody's lives, there is a greater expectation about the type, the standard and quality of that selected. I believe that, when exercising, music should not be merely bland auditory wallpaper, but that it should be appropriate, middle-of-the-road and give pleasure to the listeners. There is so much to choose from, and providing that the laws relating to copyright are observed (see below), then it is worthwhile collecting a library of suitable tapes or CDs.

Choice of Music

Whilst this is a very personal thing, there are certain guidelines that I would recommend that you follow. Music with a strong beat is better, but a solo vocal track can be distracting. If the choice is up to you, then choose something that you like. It is also preferable to have 'happy-sounding' music — and if it can make you laugh, then so much the better. For example, I find the 'Hooked on Classics' series excellent. One particular track 'A Night at the Opera', has the Hallelujah Chorus from Handel's Messiah with full choir in addition to the Royal Philharmonic Orchestra. It is so incongruous to hear this when exercising in water that it brings a smile to the face. Latin American music is also good, as is ethnic music and indeed almost anything else that you fancy, providing the rhythm is regular.

Generally speaking, the beat should be a bit slower than for equivalent dry-land exercise, but there are no firm and fast rules. Often music has an 'off' beat, or there is a double beat, so that one moves to every second beat. Usually 2/4 or 4/4 time is easier, but occasionally a slow 3/3 time waltz will fit better. Most music suitable for accompanying exercises can be broken down into 8-bar sections, which often fits well into exercise sequences with 16 repetitions.

Practical considerations

1. Acoustic difficulties

Swimming, and even hydrotherapy pools are arguably the worst possible acoustic environment.

The background noises and the echoes make it very difficult to reproduce the quality of sound that is on the recording selected. Moreover, it is necessary to talk over this cacophony of sound, in order to give instructions and deliver teaching points. Fortunately, it is not necessary to talk too much, as the slower speed of movement means that there is time to `cue' in the moves much more easily than in a non-aquatic session. Non-verbal cues are an essential part of teaching. If teaching more than a handful of people, it is necessary to project the voice, which is difficult to do without shouting. Continued voice abuse can lead to permanent voice problems by damaging the vocal chords. One solution is to be trained in the art of voice production. Another, better, solution is to use a battery-operated, hands-free microphone, preferably one that is submersible.

2. Equipment

Then there are the mechanical difficulties of the reproduction of sound. The first aspect to this concerns equipment. It is essential that only battery-operated tape/CD players be used in a pool environment. To do otherwise, even with low-voltage and circuit breakers, is contravening all health and safety guidelines. Battery machines that are designed for use in such an environment will survive longer if they can be kept dry. It is therefore sensible to keep a small hand-towel close by, to dry hands before touching the ghetto-blaster. A better solution is to have properly wired-in speakers, with an infra-red control that means it is not necessary to touch the tape-deck.

Copyright Issues

Using music during an exercise class is defined as giving a public performance. There are therefore several legal obligations that result from this. The person in charge (the coach) requires a Public Performance Licence (PPL) and so do the premises. Needless to say, licences cost money.

According to current international law, it is illegal to make copies of CDs or tapes. This means that it is against the law to compile one's own 'mix' of tapes. The interpretation of this law seems to vary in different countries. In North America, it seems to be standard practice to compile one's own mixes, as indeed used to be the practice in the UK until just a few years ago. There are two legal ways around this difficulty in the UK. One is to subscribe to a specialized musical recording company that has permission to make its own compilations, which it then sells under sublicence to coaches. The other is to purchase specially made tapes which do not come under the auspices of the PPL. Both options are expensive, and seem to me to take away the basic right of the coach to select the music they want and need to use to carry out their job. After all, the price of tapes or CDs purchased in all shops includes a royalty which goes to reimburse the composers and musicians. The recording companies (who indirectly are the ones who enforce the no-copying law) presumably make their money directly from sales. So this restriction on compiling from tapes/CDs that you personally own (even if you do not intend to sell or lease the compilation that you have personally made) seems grossly unfair.

You will soon reach a *modus vivendi* with those distracting legal issues. So, armed with the right music (unless, of course you can persuade live musicians to play at the pool-side), choreograph your session with enthusiasm and creativity, and make it an acoustically pleasing one for all.

Section II
Specific Population Groups

To be a good physiotherapist or fitness coach, you must enjoy interacting with people, as good communication skills are prerequisites for both professions. It is therefore likely that this next section of the book, which deals with people, will have more inherent appeal than the preceding section which is primarily concerned with the underpinning science.

Section II deals with groups of people who could broadly be classified as those who are likely to have special needs, or require special assistance. However, the concept of special need is a broad one. For example, those over 60 generally require a different exercise regime than do the young and fit; but they may themselves be fit and not require any special assistance. Moreover, it is pos-sible that the 'special needs' client population could fall into more than one of the categories dealt with in the following chapter; for example, they could be elderly and have a musculoskeletal problem. However, they are unlikely to be both elderly and pregnant.

With these caveats, physical performance as related to exercise in water, will be dealt with in terms of five separate population groups. The first two classifications are non-pathological: those people who are in the latter half of life and those who are, or have recently been, pregnant. The next three chapters are concerned with people with problems: arthritis, orthopaedic con-ditions and obesity, which in itself is not a prob-lem, but which is a predisposing factor to disease.

6

Aquarobics for Later life

What is Later Life?

At this point, a definition of later life would be appropriate, but it is difficult to be precise. The concept of 'who is elderly' is not only subjective, but appears to vary according to cultural and national mores. Some years ago, one would have referred to 'senior citizens' or possibly 'pensioners', and meant it to apply to those aged about 65 or older. However, political correctness has now outlawed the use of such terms, whilst in the UK, for example, the average age for retirement (or irreversible 'redundancy') has lowered considerably. In parallel, the chronological benchmark in public health definitions of later life has also lowered to encompass all people over the age of 50. It is interesting that as life expectancy has increased, and the discrepancy in many individuals between 'functional' (biological) and chronological age has widened, so the official watershed for entering 'later life' has decreased. One effect of this is that this 'mature' section of society now accounts for about 50% of the UK population. I am in the latter part of that demicentury decade, but feel young, work-out regularly and am more productive than I have ever been. With a bit of luck, and some planning, I hope to have my health and strength for another 20–30 years. (That is not unrealistic, a surprising percentage of 80+ year olds still live extremely active lives (HMSO, 1996).)

The World Health Organization (WHO) 'Heidelberg' Guidelines for Promoting Physical Activity among Older Persons states that 'Age 50 marks a point in middle age at which the benefits of regular physical activity can be most relevant in avoiding, minimizing, and/or reversing many of the physical, psychological, and social hazards which often accompany advancing age. These beneficial effects apply to most individuals regardless of health status and/or disease state.' The WHO policy is to encourage active exercise participation for people aged over 50, and many countries now have such programmes. The health benefits are indisputable (Aniansson et al., 1984; Morey et al., 1991; Campbell et al., 1997).

Aquatic exercise has a special role for those in later life. The earlier chapters in this book have elaborated the reasons for the beneficial effects of aquatic exercise regardless of age. However, those in later years are more vulnerable to adverse effects of land-based exercise than are those in their forties or younger. Many of the hazards associated with exercise, such as 'wear and tear' on joints, falling over or colliding, are more likely to have serious sequelae in the older population, and such people are more likely to fall over than the young in the first place because of the various physiological changes that tend to happen with increasing age. In the water, it is not normally dangerous to fall over, the risk of joint injury is minimal because of the lack of weight-bearing and the risk of intrinsic muscle damage is very small. All in all, aquatic exercise for the elderly could be said to give the gain without the pain or the hazard.

The Ageing Process

The ageing process is characterized by a deterioration in the function of some or all of the body's systems. An attractive current theory is that it may be caused by bio-energy loss due to accumulated somatic oxidative damage to mitochondrial DNA, the rate of which may, in part, be genetically determined (Linnane *et al.*, 1989). Whatever the mechanism it will be many years before the process is not only understood but can be postponed or prevented. Nonetheless, this last 50 years has seen major increases in life expectancy in many Western countries. Current issues are concerned with the quality of this extended life, and the possible role of aquatic exercise in helping to improve this.

The main anatomical and physiological changes that can take place with advancing years, and the implication of such changes for aquatic exercise, are discussed below. However, whether or not such changes take place, and at what rate is uncertain and variable. There are many octogenarians who are younger in 'outlook' and others who can produce greater physical performances than people half their age. The science underlying ageing is being investigated in many major laboratories around the world. This is not merely because it is one of the great unsolved problems of biology, and of great humanitarian significance. It is also of personal interest to all scientists (who like most people would like to live longer and stay healthy). Immense rewards, both commercial and in terms of prestige and honour, will be heaped on the persons or organizations that can delay or mitigate the ageing process.

There are many different kinds of tissue that make up the human body. Most of these are subject to degeneration linked with age. The resultant changes have implications for Aquarobics classes. The implications for each tissue will now be examined.

Skin

The changes to the skin that normally accompany age are perhaps the most obvious, as skin is the most visible and extensive organ of the body. The actual make up of skin varies with different parts of the body, and according to usage; for example, the eyelid is much thinner than the soles of the feet. Although such differences are primarily genetic, there is leeway for environmental adaptation: for example, manual workers will develop thicker skin on their hands than sedentary workers.

All skin contains specialist cells, such as blood and lymph vessels, nerves, sweat glands and hair follicles, but these are contained within a double-sheeted matrix (Thomson *et al.*, 1991). The outer sheet, the multi-layered **epidermis** is characterized by its stratum corneum, a relatively thick layer of dead cells which makes a hard, waterproof outer surface made from the protein keratin. This changes very little with age. However, the other layers of the epidermis do change with age, so that the whole epidermis becomes thinner and the number of specialized cells within it are diminished. The underlying *dermis* also thins (by about 20%) with age and the number of specialist cells within it also declines. Alteration in collagen and elastic tissue in the dermis lead to the skin becoming less resilient and elastic, and more wrinkly. There is usually a layer of subcutaneous fat underneath the dermis. The ageing process results in this subcutaneous fat being dispersed towards the abdominal cavity.

THERMOREGULATION

The overall result of these changes is easy to see. A baby's skin is smooth and thick, whereas the skin of its grandparent will be more wrinkly, flexible and thinner. Young skin is a better insulator, not only because of its depth, but because of the layer of subcutaneous fat. Skin, containing its extensive vascular network, is the main body organ concerned with thermoregulation. Older people are therefore more prone to feeling the cold, not only because of the lack of insulation but because of the reduced (and possibly less responsive) vascular network.

This is why older people are particularly more sensitive to cool water in swimming pools. They will not only 'feel cold', but they will lose heat more quickly. Heat needs to be generated by muscular activity, so relaxation periods must be kept short, and heat loss should be limited by keeping as much of the body underwater as possible, thereby limiting cooling through the latent heat of evaporation (see Chapter 3). It may also be necessary to curtail the length of time allocated for a 'seniors' class.

The water in the average swimming pool is considerably below body temperature, and the structure of an exercise session must reflect the need for activities which will generate heat by having intensive, short bursts of exercise throughout.

The warm-up should be extended and the cooldown curtailed. Good observation of participants is necessary because the way in which the body minimizes heat loss is by shivering, and by vasoconstriction of the skin. This latter causes the skin to become very white, and if this happens on a whole-body scale, then blood pressure could rise to a potentially hazardous level.

On the other hand, if the exercise is happening in a hydrotherapy pool, at a temperature which is thermoneutral or above, then there is a danger of hyperthermia. Vasodilation will happen on a major scale, and dizziness could result, or even more serious overload stress to the cardiovascular system. Hyperthermia is more likely to happen if the clients are overweight, as the fat insulates the body core and does not permit the heat produced by exercise to be conducted away. The vascular response is often less obvious in people with a deep layer of subcutaneous fat. Again, observation is necessary. Becoming too flushed or florid is a warning sign. Sweating from the head is another. See Chapter 4 for further details.

It is therefore essential for therapists and aquatic teachers to observe their clients, and be prepared to take appropriate action, such as terminating a session for an individual or the whole group, or having cold water added to the pool if the water temperature is too high. If the pool is small, it is relatively easy to reduce the water temperature quickly (within my own clinic and pool I can easily switch on the hose). However, such apparently simple procedures are frequently impossible, because of administrative procedures, in the highly organized world of the leisure centre or hospital. If the pool is too cold, it is difficult to increase the temperature rapidly, even in a small private facility. So temperature control of the pool requires planning well in advance.

THE ABILITY TO FLOAT

There is another relevant point which comes from the loss of subcutaneous fat with ageing. The ability to float may be affected. If the fat has shifted centrally, to the abdomen, then the centre of buoyancy will have shifted anteriorly. It may make it easier to float supine on the surface, as the trunk will be more buoyant, but the loss of fat in the limbs will mean that there is less support (and possibly stability) when standing in the water. Keeping the arms down at the sides (when standing) will be easier, but lifting the arms up through abduction or flexion will require more muscle effort to compensate for the lack of buoyancy. People who 20 years earlier floated with ease may find that this redistribution of body tissues has changed their ability - for the better or worse. Care, particular observation and possibly some help may therefore be necessary the first time a new client is asked to lie supine.

A final point relevant to age-related skin changes and aquatic exercise is that older people tend to suffer from dry skin, which needs to be lubricated by creams and ointments. The use of soap can make this condition worse. Physicians sometimes advise really old people not to bathe (and use soap) more than two or three times a week. It could be that the chlorine or other chemicals in the water aggravate an underlying dry skin condition. Showering after being in the pool helps to wash away the chemicals, but perhaps it is not necessary to use soap. An information sheet about aquatic exercise could suggest to clients that they should observe their skin, in case there is any reaction to the pool water.

Muscle

There are well-documented changes to muscle tissue which happen with age (Beverley et al., 1989; Skelton et al., 1995). Several studies have shown that resistance training can increase strength, power and selected functional activities, even if such activities are not started until advanced later life, i.e. over the age of 85 (Beverley et al., 1989). Whether or not such training can be undertaken in the water is not yet scientifically established.

The key muscle groups to strengthen in later life are those which are necessary in order to maintain independence: the functional, anti-gravity extensor groups of the knee, hip and back and the calves. In addition, the biceps, the muscles of the pelvic floor and, to some extent, all of the muscular system needs to maintain a basic level of fitness that is appropriate to age and lifestyle.

Muscle injuries are probably rarer in older people, apart from complete ruptures of the biceps. This is probably due to a weakening or reduction in the quantity and quality of the connective tissues, thereby making the attachments of the muscle vulnerable. It is therefore probably a sensible precaution to plan exercises so that there is a gradual increase in fibre recruitment rather than a sudden all-out effort. As there is normally no warning when the biceps ruptures, it could be argued that this would be going to happen in any case. The author has not heard of an instance when the long head of biceps has been ruptured whilst exercising in the pool but, theoretically, this could happen — even while swimming. Examples of appropriate exercises which will enhance muscle performance in later life can be found in Section IV.

When muscles are put through a training programme, there is an increase in gross muscle strength and power, as measured in functional tests and by various histological parameters, such as an increase in the number and size of fibres (please refer to Chapters 2 and 12). The benefits are also felt beyond the muscular system, in the skeleton itself, and result in an enhanced composition of bone.

Bone

The composition of bone is highly complex. Bone is a type of connective tissue consisting of organic material such as collagen and mineral salts, calcium, magnesium and phosphorus. The first provides the resilience whilst the others provide the strength and support. Throughout life, bone is continually being structured and broken down, and in order to achieve this state of 'plasticity' there needs to be a balance between osteoblasts and osteoclasts – the cells which respectively build and break down bone. Some degree of bone loss is an inevitable sequelae of the ageing process, and this is usually because of a reduction in the number and efficiency of osteoblasts. However, the whole process is highly complicated and depends on the absorption and manufacture of vitamin D, the supply of minerals such as calcium and correct hormone control.

Osteoporosis is a disease characterized by micro-architectural deterioration of bone tissue leading to low bone mass (WHO, 1994). Osteomalacia is a condition in which the bone has a lower mineral content. Both conditions are liable to result in fractures. Some 22% of a group of 241 patients whose average age was 75 had died within a year of fracturing their hip (White *et al.*, 1987). Vertebral fractures in the elderly are a major cause of pain, deformity and distress. The third common site of fractures is the wrist, and although less serious medically, the enforced inactivity can cause major functional problems. Some of the deleterious results of osteoporosis can be mitigated by weight-bearing exercise, correct diet (including vitamin D supplement), and drugs aimed at the hormone control or calcium metabolism.

The most important aim of prophylactic exercise for osteoporosis is to reduce the rate of bone loss. This can be done by weight-bearing activities and body resistance strength training. As the hip and the vertebrae are weight-bearing regions, the accepted practice is to encourage weight-bearing exercise. Certainly it appears that strong muscle work is necessary to achieve the desired effect. A study showed that squeezing a ball hard for 30 seconds a day, for 6 weeks, brought about a significant increase in grip strength and bone mineral content, thereby suggesting that it is the size of the muscle contraction and not merely the weight-bearing (Beverley *et al.*, 1989). As vertical exercise in the water is largely non-weight-bearing, there is debate as to whether it can be beneficial in preventing fractures in osteoporosis. There has been no study showing any evidence of improved bone density through aquatic exercise. To be effective, it would be necessary to perform fairly strong resistance exercises in the water in order to work muscles sufficiently hard to minimize bone loss. Such a study needs to be done. There are other effects of water exercise, such as improvements in muscle strength, aerobic power and balance (Simmons and Hansen, 1996), and the reduction of pain. The improvement in balance should help to reduce the risk of falls which might result in fractures. A recent study in New Zealand (Campbell *et al.*, 1997) showed that the risk of falls in women aged over 80 could be significantly reduced by having them undertake an exercise programme that included balance. This can certainly be achieved in the water (see below).

Joints

Joints are complex junctions. They are microcosmic environments with their own circulation and nerve supply, all encapsulated in a sheath. Like all other tissues, joints are prone to changes with age. There are, of course, specific diseases of joints – inflammatory, infective and autoimmune, and these are known as various types of arthropathy (or arthritis). The most common of these is osteoarthritis, also known as degenerative arthritis or just 'wear-and-tear'. It is difficult to know how much of this is an exaggeration or exacerbation of the normal ageing process (possibly precipitated by trauma many years earlier) and how much is a separate disease process. Almost everybody over the age of 35 has some 'wear and tear' changes in their spine, as confirmed by X-rays. However, only a small percentage of this population will complain of pain or malfunction in these same joints. There are yet others who appear to demonstrate the clinical signs of osteoarthritis, in the spine, hips or knees, but whose X-rays are normal.

Chapter 8 deals further with arthritis, but since osteoarthritis is associated so strongly with age, some overlap here is unavoidable. The implications of aquatic exercise for older people with minor joint dysfunctions will be considered here; those with acute or more serious pathology will be covered in Chapter 8. Details of the changes that occur in and around joint tissues will also be left until Chapter 8.

There are several advantages of aquatic (as opposed to conventional) exercise for older people with minor degenerative joint disease.

1. Buoyancy dramatically reduces the weight being transmitted through damaged and painful articular cartilage and other sensitive joint tissues (see Chapter 3). Exercise is therefore likely to be much less painful, and so a lot more fun.
2. The ability to move fast through the water allows for the possibility of aerobic exercise like running, and possibly even jumping – activities that might be prevented by pain when not immersed. This means that an aquatic work-out is probably more effective when looked at from an overall fitness perspective.
3. The release of endorphins, which is facilitated by exercise of moderate intensity, will help to reduce pain and produce a sense of well-being, which will outlast the exercise for several hours or possibly longer.
4. The degenerative process appears to be modified by pain-free movement: and this is a genuine therapeutic and even more long-lasting effect.

So are there any special precautions or adaptations that are required by this group of people? Most importantly, the water should be chest high to provide enough buoyancy to produce weight relief. If the pool is too shallow, it may be necessary to sit on stools, or adapt the exercises so that there is minimum weight-bearing. The other important factor is water temperature. Generally speaking, chronically malfunctioning older joints perform better if they do not get too cold. It is therefore preferable to be in water that is tepid.

Urinary System

An important function of the kidneys is to monitor and maintain the normal balance of water and body salt, as well as to filter out and excrete water-soluble toxins and waste products. With age, the kidneys become smaller and filter less blood (Williams, 1995). These changes increase the possibility of damage to them by toxins or diseases, but unless they are so affected, ageing kidneys usually continue to function adequately, if less efficiently, into extreme old age. As mentioned in Chapter 3, vertical immersion is likely to reduce unwanted fluid in interstitial tissues, such as that found in cases of mild heart or renal failure, the mechanism for this being the central fluid redistribution modulated by the increase in hydrostatic pressure, and the resultant 700% increase in diuresis (urine production). To rephrase this into non-technical jargon, vertical immersion combined with gentle exercise, can reduce dramatically the surplus fluid which gathers in certain medical conditions.

Incontinence of urine is not uncommon in the older population. It can often be helped by pelvic floor strengthening exercises (which will be explained in greater detail in Chapter 7). Ideally, such exercises should be included in any health-related exercise class for this age group. In fact, it seems particularly appropriate to practice when immersed in a pool.

A practical consideration is the availability of toilet facilities. A small leakage of urine (which is sterile under normal circumstances) does not cause any public health hazard to other pool occupants, particularly if pool filtration and disinfection are maintained at recommended levels. It is, though a social embarrassment if spotted. All clients should be advised to void their bladders before getting into the pool, and should know where the nearest lavatory is situated — ideally very close by. (Any faecal contamination into pool water is a hazard and is incompatible with pool immersion.)

Cardiovascular and Respiratory Systems

Although it is very common to have changes in the heart muscle, heart valves, the coronary blood supply and the cells that control the timing of the heart beat, it is probable that the more serious of these are the result of disease process and not simply the passing of time. Changes that probably are due to the ageing process are an alteration in the elastic properties of heart muscle, prolonged contraction time, increased resistance to electrical stimulation and a reduced response to certain cardiac medication. The blood vessels are also prone to age-related change: the connective tissue in the large arteries becomes thickened and the cells lining the blood vessels are prone to irregularities (Williams, 1995).

The cardiovascular system responds less efficiently to various stresses with age. The maximum heart rate, which is approximately 220 minus age, must therefore reduce by one beat a year, and hence the training heart rate will also get lower. The resting heart rate and the cardiac output do not change. Any age-related changes in heart rate on exercise will, however, be masked by the reduction of about 10 beats a minute that occurs on immersion.

The trachea and the large airways increase in diameter as we age, but there is a reduction in the surface area of actual lung tissue. Lung elasticity decreases, leading to an increase in lung volume. The chest expands and the diaphragm descends. The ribs can become less mobile, and this can increase the work demand on the respiratory muscles. The functional outcome of these physical changes is that vital capacity declines linearly between the ages of 20 and 80. The amount of residual air left after expiration increases from about 20% at the age of 20 to 35% at the age of 60. There is also a reduction in the amount of oxygen dissolved in the blood. Age does not affect the ability to dispose of carbon dioxide (Williams, 1995).

The conclusion appears to be that respiratory function tends to deteriorate with age. However, this effect can be counteracted if endurance training is undertaken; this can lead to dramatic improvements in aerobic capacity. However, a potential hazard is that those individuals who may have mild respiratory impairment just below the threshold of producing clinical signs when undertaking moderate exercise on dry land, may get too breathless when exercising immersed, because of the hydrostatic pressure exerting an additional force on the chest wall.

The Neurological System

Nerve cells in the brain and spinal cord are one of the few tissues in the body that do not regenerate. With ageing, there is a loss of these neurons in the grey matter, the cerebellum and the hippocampus. This latter is probably associated with memory loss. In some cases, the neurons survive, but the density of their interconnections becomes diminished. There is, though, a slow, continued growth in synapses (nerve connections), which suggest a continual re-patterning or plasticity of connections. There is a decline of brain proteins, particularly of some enzymes and some abnormal proteins are produced. The blood supply to the brain decreases between 15 and 20% between the ages of 30 and 70. It is possible that this reduced blood supply mediates some of the other changes (Williams, 1995).

Intellectual function, language skills, the ability to concentrate and behaviour are probably not affected by the above structural changes. Probably the first deterioration that can be blamed on age is in the ability to retain large amounts of knowledge over a long period of time. There is no inevitability about any of these changes and there are very many old people who can outperform those who are much younger, particularly if they keep themselves intellectually stimulated.

Although intellectual function need not deteriorate with ageing, other integrative functions of the brain may become compromised. This is particularly the case with balance. The mechanism of balance is very complex. It involves many neurological pathways including reflex arcs and sensory (proprioceptive) impulses from specialized nerve endings around joints and in muscles, all of which are monitored by the higher centres, which respond by sending impulses to muscles to cause the movements necessary to prevent falling over. It really is an extremely complicated but wonderfully efficient system. Like everything else in the body, it needs to be used or it ceases to be as efficient, but it is never too late to retrain. The opposite scenario is a complete loss of confidence, involving hanging on to furniture, walls or walking aids — all of which lead to further degeneration in balance function.

The way to improve balance is to have the body taken to the point of falling over, but then to make the necessary adaptation to regain stability. This is a dangerous exercise in the home because it is too easy to misjudge, and fall. However, balance exercises can take place in the pool, as the viscosity of the water slows down the toppling process, giving an opportunity to make correction. If the worst comes to the worst, a few hops or a mild ducking are safer than risking falls on hard ground. Exercises standing on one leg whilst moving the centre of gravity without falling over, are all extremely helpful and may prevent subsequent falls at home, leading to serious fractures. Woggles and floats can be used to help retrain balance. For example sitting on a woggle, as on a swing, and balancing.

In addition to instinctive balance, coordination too can be improved in the water by putting together a few movements to make an easy short routine, which can be repeated. This encourages learning, memory and coordination. Routines, though, must be kept very short and simple initially.

Table 6.1
Effects of ageing and implications for Aquarobics

Tissue	Change	Implications for aqua-exercise
Skin	Loss of collagen, elasticity and subcutaneous fat	Risk of getting chilled in the water
Muscle	Reduction in number and size of fibres	Deterioration in strength: reversible with strength training
Bone	Reduction in mineral content: osteoporosis	Lessened by strong muscle contraction
Joints	Degenerative arthritis	Easier movement in the water, ? difficulty getting dressed and pool access
Urinary system	Possible poor sphincter control	May require nearby WC
Cardiovascular and pulmonary systems	Possible pathology affecting ability to exercise	Careful screening and observation for (gentle) aerobic training
Neurological system (a) Coordination (b) Memory and intellect (c) The five senses	Poor balance, ? difficulty with learning 'moves', ? visual or hearing difficulties	Do balance training, simple moves, many repetitions, careful positioning and choice of music

Vision, hearing and smell deteriorate markedly with age, whereas taste and touch, the other two senses may only become somewhat less sensitive. When planning an aquatic class for those in later life, it must be remembered that the participants need to be able to see the teacher, and must therefore be close by. Glasses can be worn for Aquarobics, but care is required. The risk of not seeing properly is probably greater than the risk of losing the glasses — providing they fit well. It is useful to have a dry cloth to hand at the poolside, in case the lenses get splashed.

Poor hearing is more of a problem. Firstly, the acoustics are always bad in swimming pools — and they are made worse by the use of music. Secondly, hearing aids should not be worn in the water as they can get lost or irrevocably damaged. Those with impaired vision or hearing should be positioned close to the teacher.

Summary

It is daunting to have written so much about the problems of getting old, especially as most people aspire to live to a ripe old age, enjoying as full a life as possible. For there is a truly positive side to later life: not only the well-earned leisure and opportunity to explore new interests and experiences, but the enjoyment and fulfilment that comes through having an extended (and, hopefully, extending) circle of family and friends. The only fear is that one hopes not to become a burden. The evidence is now very strong that participation in exercise is likely to diminish the possibility of becoming a burden, by maintaining independence. Aquatic exercise is a particularly appropriate way in which to exercise in the latter part of life.

References

Aniansson A, Ljungberg P, Runddgren A and Wetterqvist H (1984) Effect of a training programme for pensioners on condition and muscular strength. *Arch Gerontol Geriatr* 3(3): 229–241.

Beverley MC, Rider TA, Evans MJ and Smith R (1989) Local bone mineral response to brief exercise that stresses the skeleton. *Br Med J* **299**: 233–235.

Campbell AJ, Robertson MC, Gardner MM *et al.* (1997) Randomised controlled trial of a general practice programme of home based exercise to prevent falls in elderly women. *Br Med J* **315**: 1065–1069.

HMSO (1996) *Getting Around After 60: A Profile of Britain's Older Population.* HMSO, London.

Linnane AW, Marzuki S, Ozawa T and Tanaka M (1989) Mitochondrial DNA mutations as an important contributor to ageing and degenerative diseases. *Lancet* i: 642–645.

Morey MC, Cowper PA, Foussner JR *et al.* (1991) Two-year trends in physical performance following supervised exercise among community-dwelling older veterans. *J Am Geriatr Soc* **39**(6): 549–554.

Simmons V and Hansen PD (1996) Effectiveness of water exercise on postural mobility in well elderly: An experimental study on balance enhancement. *J Gerontol* **51A**(5): M233–238.

Skelton DA, Young A, Greig CA and Malbut KE (1995) Effects of resistance training on strength, power, and selected functional abilities of women aged 75 and older. *J Am Geriatr Soc* **43**: 1081–1087.

Thomson A, Skinner A and Piercy J (eds) (1991) *Tidy's Physiotherapy*, ch. 17. Butterworth-Heinemann, London.

White BL, Fisher WD and Laurin CA (1987) Rate of mortality for elderly patients after fracture of the hip in the 1980s. *J Bone Joint Surg* **69**(9): 1335–1340.

Williams ME (1995) *Complete Guide to Aging and Health.* Harmony Books, New York, p. 387.

World Health Organization (1994) *Assessment of Fracture Risk and its Application to Screening for Postmenopausal Osteoporosis.* Report of a WHO Study group; WHO technical report series 843. WHO, Geneva.

World Health Organization (1996) *The Heidelberg Guidelines for Promoting Physical Activity among Older People.* Guidelines Series for Healthy Aging - I. WHO, Geneva.

7

Before and After Childbirth

Pregnancy is not a disease, but a perfectly normal physiological state, and many women of child-bearing age are accustomed to exercise and choose to continue throughout their pregnancy. However, if there are any complications in the pregnancy, leading to an increased risk of miscarriage, or if the pregnancy is of twins (or more), then even moderate exercise, including aquatics, is not appropriate. On the other hand, if all is normal, then exercise is helpful, and water is the ideal medium for this. In later pregnancy, women are sometimes heard to complain that they feel like whales. Think how gracefully and effortlessly whales move in the water!

The Benefits of Exercise When Pregnant

There is a growing body of literature suggesting that moderate aquatic exercise during pregnancy is helpful to both mother and baby. Wallace *et al.* (1986), Wallace and Engstron (1987) and Katz *et al.* (1991) were in favour of moderate aerobic exercise during pregnancy as it led to less complications during pregnancy and childbirth, higher maternal self-esteem and lower discomfort during the last trimester. Zeanah and Schlosser (1993) undertook a survey of 173 aerobically-orientated women to see if they were familiar with, and conformed to, the American College of Obstetrics and Gynecology (ACOG) Guidelines limiting dry-land exercise to a maximum heart rate of 140 beats a minute for 20 minutes. 53% were aware of the guidelines, but many of them admitted to exercising at a greater intensity than that recommended. There were no significant differences in maternal weight gain, fetal birthweight or gestational age of the newborn, between those that exercised moderately and more excessively. However, the women in the study who did adhere to the ACOG guidelines had significantly fewer Caesarean deliveries.

With regard to aquatics, Katz (1991) found that aquatic exercise had less effect on fetal cardiovascular parameters than land exercise of similar intensity. But whether or not there are specific physiological benefits from doing so, pregnant women report enjoying exercising in water as it feels appropriate. The buoyancy of the water removes the extra weight from overworked ligaments and joints, and this sensation is recognized and appreciated by the participants. In the UK the growth of antenatal and postnatal classes in swimming and hydrotherapy pools has been dramatic, and it is to be hoped that the many women participating do find some benefit from them.

Why Not Simply Swim?

It is better to exercise-to-music in water when pregnant than to swim because the latter can strain the already taxed lumbar spine. One of the complications of pregnancy is low back pain, often due to the extra weight of the uterus and the baby on ligaments, particularly those around the sacroiliac joints. The typical pregnant posture is to overextend the lumbar spine to compensate for the centre of gravity which has moved forward. (Postural advice should be given to correct this, and such advice can, of course, be delivered in the water just as easily as on land.) To return to swimming, breast stroke (most women's favourite stroke) tends to increase lumbar extension, and can therefore exacerbate a backache. In fact, it is not only the back, but all joints in the body that are vulnerable to overstretching during pregnancy because of lax ligaments. The knees are also particularly vulnerable and can be injured by breast stroke. Relaxin, a hormone secreted during early pregnancy, causes ligaments which are normally inelastic to stretch, in order to make more space within the mother's body for the baby. Ligaments remain lengthened until about five months after the baby is born. To prevent injury, all exercise when pregnant should be within a comfortable range of movement and should not attempt to mobilize joints.

Physiological Changes of Pregnancy

Body Fat

In addition to the change modulated by relaxin, there are many other modifications to the maternal body during pregnancy. One of the first changes to occur is an increase in body fat. This probably has evolutionary significance in that the fat is a potential source of nourishment for mother and baby in times of hardship or famine. Because fat has a lower specific gravity than other tissues, it will be easier for a pregnant woman to float. Moreover, her centre of gravity might now be different than before, so she will need to re-learn how to maintain a balanced posture when exercising standing in water.

Increased body fat also makes a pregnant woman at risk of hyperthermia when working hard in warm water.

Cardiovascular Changes and Training

The cardiovascular changes in pregnancy are extremely significant. By the end of the first trimester, there is an increase in plasma volume of about 50%, and cardiac output rises by 40%. This is partly due to an increase in heart size. There is therefore absolutely no need for a pregnant women to exercise at training intensities, as the presence of a growing baby is already doing this to her body. The ACOG recommendations for dry-land exercise are that the heart rate should not exceed 140 beats per minute. In the water, the heart rate will be lowered by the effect of hydrostatic pressure (see Chapter 3). A lower target heart rate of 130 beats per minute should therefore be the maximum achieved during Aquarobics.

There are close similarities between cardiovascular changes that occur normally during pregnancy and when taking part in an aerobic training programme.

Possible Teratogenic Effects of Exercise in the First Trimester

It could potentially be hazardous to the mother and baby to work with the heart rate at too high an intensity, particularly early on in pregnancy, as there is some evidence that an increase in core temperature can damage the developing fetus (McMurray and Katz, 1990; Sternfeld, 1997). Exercise at a training intensity of 70% maximum can increase core body temperature, especially in the less fit, which is probably why urine feels hot when passing water after a hard 'work-out'. As indicated above, the increase in body fat during pregnancy may amplify such effects.

It should be emphasized that this potential damage to the growing embryo is a risk of the first trimester of pregnancy. By 16 weeks of gestation the embryo is fully formed, albeit very small. It is possible that any damage to the embryo could happen before the woman even knows that she is pregnant. Perhaps it would be wise for all fitness coaches to warn their female class members that they should not work at intensities over 65% VO_2 if there is a possibility that they may be pregnant.

Renal Effects

The glomerular filtration rate increases by 40–60% during pregnancy. In Chapter 3, it was seen that immersion also leads to an increase in glomerular filtration. This additional filtration may be of benefit in the late stages of pregnancy, when swelling around the ankles is not uncommon (especially in hot weather). It is advisable to encourage participants to drink before, during and after a pool session, and it should therefore be suggested that a drink be brought to the pool-side, in an unbreakable container.

Respiratory Changes

As the pregnancy progresses, the baby growing within the uterus takes up all available space within the mother's body, and pushes the abdominal contents upwards on to the diaphragm, which then elevates by up to 4 centimetres. However, this apparent loss in lung volume is compensated for by an increase in the transverse diameter of the chest, the net result of these two changes leaving the volume of the thoracic cavity unchanged (Berry *et al.*, 1989). Other studies are conflicting on the question of whether vital capacity remains the same or increases. Cugell *et al.* (1953) and Gee *et al.* (1967) found that vital capacity remained the same during pregnancy, whereas Knuttgen and Emerson (1974) found it increased. There was, however, agreement that inspiratory capacity increases during pregnancy whilst expiratory volume decreases.

The above findings illustrate changes in lung function due to pregnancy, but it must be remembered that there are also changes during immersion because of the hydrostatic pressure on the chest wall. Theoretically, a women towards the end of her pregnancy might find it a little harder to breathe if the chest is immersed. This is another reason for only exercising at a low intensity. This problem could be alleviated by moving to shallower water, so that the lungs are not immersed. Unfortunately, by so doing, some of the benefits of weightlessness on the other body tissues would be lost.

Musculoskeletal Changes

The lengthening of ligaments that results from the release of relaxin is the main change that occurs to the musculoskeletal system during pregnancy. This allows the ribs to expand transversely, as mentioned above, and the sacroiliac joints to glide open. These changes are similar to the movement which happens at the hinges of an expandable suitcase, and they create space for the growing baby within the mother's torso. Relaxin, though, is systemic in its effect, and the laxity in ligaments puts all joints in the body at greater risk of injury. Large scale dynamic exercises could take a joint beyond its normal range of movement, and are therefore contraindicated. On the other hand, muscle stretching is probably appropriate and acceptable after resistance training, providing it is slow and gentle.

Squatting is a contraindicated exercise on dry land. However, the squatting posture, or variations of it, is a common way in which women choose to deliver their babies, especially in developing countries. Squatting in the water does not create the forces produced on dry land, and is not therefore hazardous and should be incorporated into an aquatic exercise programme to 'prepare' for the birth. However, care must be taken to do this slowly and gently so as not to compromise the knee joints.

Aims of Antenatal Exercise

Enhanced Well-being

Probably the most important reason for aquatic antenatal exercise is enjoyment. It provides an opportunity for pleasurable exercise in a socially supportive context, and probably relieves some of the symptoms of discomfort which are common in later pregnancy, such as backache or swollen ankles. In the water the extra tissue gained (particularly the fat) provides additional buoyancy. Reference has already been made to a pregnant women feeling like a whale, but in water the freedom to move in any direction and sensation of being light and agile is very pleasurable. Anyone who has taken an Aquarobics class for pregnant women will have observed the look of dismay that happens as the women climb out of the water at the end of the class, and feel their 'weight' returning.

Strengthening Muscles Through Resistance Exercises

The muscles which maintain the body in a vertical posture against gravity have to work much harder to support the increased weight of the woman, the baby and all its 'baggage' (the enlarged uterus, placenta and amniotic fluid). There is an increase in weight during pregnancy of between 8 and 25 kg (Katz, 1991). It is true that the muscles are being put through a natural strengthening programme, simply by having to perform normal functional activities as the weight increases, but it is still wise to strengthen those muscle groups as part of a structured class. The leg and trunk muscles that require to be strengthened are the quadriceps, the calves, the gluteals and the back extensors. As well as these, the arm and upper trunk muscles will need to cope with the demands of motherhood after the birth, and this will involve a lot of lifting over the next two years or so. A lot of equipment is used for babies, such as car seats, carrycots and pushchairs: the safe handling of them requires strength and skill.

The muscle group that is most traumatized by normal childbirth are the muscles of the pelvic floor. Incontinence (hopefully temporary) is a not uncommon result of such trauma. Fourteen percent of women over the age of 30 suffer significant urinary leakage; trauma during childbirth and inadequate retraining thereafter is by far the most important cause. A baby's exit during a normal birth stretches the muscles of the pelvic floor, which is usually unable to function properly for a few days. It is difficult to relearn control immediately after birth, when traumatized, and the accepted practice is to teach control during pregnancy. In fact, the trauma is not only due to the birth itself; the pelvic floor is already under additional pressure during the later stages of pregnancy because the increased weight of the abdominal contents (including the baby) presses down on to the perineum. Every antenatal exercise session should include pelvic floor strengthening exercises, as it is much easier to learn the correct technique before the pressures increase. Details of how to teach pelvic floor exercises can be found on page 202. It is important to work both fast and slow fibres. Muscles are composed of both types of fibres, and each require specific exercise routines.

Out of the water, lying in the supine position is not recommended during the second half of pregnancy because the weight of the baby and the uterus pressing downwards on the inferior vena cava can cause maternal dizziness and may reduce placental blood flow. However, in the water the upward force of buoyancy counteracts this. If a floating, supine, pregnant woman bends up her knees, as though doing a reverse abdominal curl, the intra-abdominal forces will be a fraction of those produced doing the same movement on dry land, and the movement occurs without strain; the bottom simply lowers in the water as the knees are bent up. This is therefore not a contraindicated aquatic exercise.

Nonetheless, the abdominal muscle groups should not be worked hard when they are in such a weakened stretched state. Some of the gentler abdominal exercises such as Pancake Tucks (Section IV, Exercise 30) can be adapted so that they are done gently and without effort. The legs can be brought into a partial squat position so as not to interfere with the 'bump' that is the baby, and there should be no strain as the water supports the weight of the body. The one abdominal muscle which can be exercised at all times, albeit gently, is abdominis transversis. This is done by trying to pull in the tummy. It is obviously impossible to pull in the 'bump', but the muscle can still work a little by going through the motion and tensing. This muscle is very important in getting correct control to improve posture, as there is a tendency during pregnancy to increase the lumbar lordosis (Fig. 7.1). Pulling the tummy in and trying to flatten the lumbar spine is a good exercise, and should be done in all positions from standing to supine to kneeling or squatting.

Figure 7.1   Posture in pregnancy: (a) poor; (b) good.

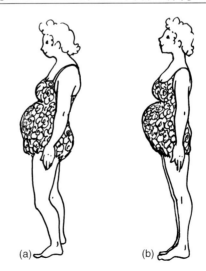

(a)   (b)

Enhancing Fitness Through Moderate Aerobic Exercise

It has already been stated that only mild to moderate aerobic exercises should be performed, as those of greater intensity are unnecessary and possibly harmful. Nonetheless, mild aerobic exercise can be performed in shoulder-high water, without the risk of damage to otherwise overloaded tissues. Such exercise may release endorphins, which will further enhance the beneficial effect of the exercise. It must be remembered that the American College of Obstetrics and Gynecology (ACOG, 1994) guideline for exercise during pregnancy (Appendix 7.1), needs to be modified for aquatic use. It is therefore suggested that 130 beats a minute would be a more appropriate target for aquatic exercise, and that this intensity should not be maintained for more than 15 minutes. Moreover, pregnant women over the age of 30 should perhaps reduce their target rate still further, as this target is age-related. Probably it is wiser to forget about heart rate altogether, and use the Borg RPE Scale (see Table 7.1) and aim for a level between weak and moderate (2–3).

Muscle Stretching Through Flexibility Exercises

As already stated, pregnancy is not a time to work at joint flexibility because lax ligaments may allow movement beyond the normal range and damage could result. However, there is no reason why muscle stretching exercises should not be performed to those muscle groups which have been worked while in the water. The muscle groups which may require stretching are the calf, the quadriceps, the hamstrings, the biceps and the triceps (see Section IV, muscle stretches).

Gentle, slow squatting, either on the floor of the pool if shallow enough, or against the pool wall (providing there is something to hold on to) is a useful preparation for childbirth and an exercise which feels good and natural. However, care must be taken not to force the abducted position, as it strains the symphysis pubis joint, a dysfunction of which is a complication of pregnancy.

Relaxation

Learning to relax is a normal part of preparation for childbirth. Floating, with the support of buoyant objects such as woggles, is an excellent way to practise this, providing the water is warm enough. Without using buoyant objects, it is generally impossible to float with rigid limbs and unsupported floating therefore requires relaxation. Being slowly propelled through the water whilst floating, and feeling the water moving against one's skin, is a pleasurable and relaxing activity. This is perhaps best done in couples - one person floating and the other supporting them and moving them around. It is the perfect way to terminate an exercise session if the water is warm enough. Shivering is incompatible with relaxation!

Precautions

Aquatic exercise *per se*, during pregnancy is inherently very safe. There are, though, some rare complications of pregnancy which, if present, mean that exercise is contraindicated. Table 7.2 below lists those contraindications.

A hydrotherapy pool may be too warm for pregnant women to exercise in — hyperthermia is a possibility. Conversely, if the water is too cold, then vasoconstriction in the legs could theoretically cause an increase in blood pressure. Careful observation is necessary to ensure that nobody is getting too warm or too cold.

Table 7.1
Summary of the aims of aquatic exercise in pregnancy

Aim	Action
Enjoyment	A well-planned, interesting session to likeable music
Muscle strengthening and posture correction	Work anti-gravity muscles of legs and trunk, arm muscles and pelvic floor
Aerobic fitness	Low intensity only
Flexibility	No joint stretching. Only gentle stretching of the muscles that have been strengthened
Relaxation	Floating, if the water is warm enough

Table 7.2
Contraindication for exercise during pregnancy requiring medical intervention

Condition	Symptoms
Hypertension caused by the pregnancy	Sudden swelling of the ankles, hands or face, headaches, visual disturbance, dizziness, sudden severe upper abdominal pain
History of miscarriage or premature labour	Vaginal bleeding; ruptured membranes
Low-weight baby Multiple pregnancy	Possibly insufficient weight gain
Excessive fatigue, chest pain, palpitations	
Unexplained abdominal pain or uterine contractions	
Phlebitis	Swelling, pain or redness in the calf of one leg

The Aquarobics principles should be observed at all times, and observing them should prevent awkward movements, such as extending the leg too far behind, which can strain the lumbar spine, or indeed doing any excessive joint movement. It is important to screen adequately beforehand, and make sure that the participants know they must stop at any time if they do not feel well, or have any pain.

Table 7.3
Summary of precautions necessary for antenatal aquatic exercise

Potential hazard	Result	Preventive action
Water too warm	Hyperthermia; feeling faint or dizzy	Reduce exercise intensity
Water too cold	Hypothermia; possible increase in blood pressure	Increase exercise intensity and/or curtail session
Over-vigorous leg abduction	Symphysis pubis dysfunction	Avoid all exercises with vigorous, dynamic leg ad- or abduction, e.g. star jumps
Vigorous toe pointing	Cramp	Avoid the activity
Large dynamic movements	Possible joint damage	Gentle, small-range movements

Ensure that participants have good breast support: this may be better obtained by wearing a normal bra and T-shirt than an unsupportive swimming costume. Enlarged breasts will float and bras therefore need support from above and below! Activities such as jumping (which would otherwise be safe in shoulder-high water) will cause a drag on the breasts. It may be better to work in shoulder-depth water, which will allow the breasts to float, rather than low chest-height where the surface tension would drag the breasts down. Similarly, avoid jumping high out of the water as the surface tension will drag the breasts down and landing will place some force through the vulnerable joints of the spine and pelvis.

Common discomforts of pregnancy include backache and muscular cramps. It has already been stated that gentle lumbar movements may assist reduction in backache, and so such movements should be included in an aquatic programme. However, other movements such as strong pointing of the toes can precipitate cramp in the muscles of the lower leg and should therefore be avoided.

Postnatal Exercise

When Can Aquatic Exercise Start?

Dry-land exercise activities such as aerobics should not be started until at least six weeks after giving birth because weight-bearing exercise through vulnerable, recovering joints can be hazardous, and weakened muscles like the pelvic floor or the abdominals could be damaged. It is possible, however, to start Aquarobics sooner because such hazardous forces do not exist when immersed. It is not advisable to participate in Aquarobics until the perineum is properly healed and any discharge has ceased. Moreover, some pools are overloaded with chlorine or other chemicals, and these could damage the sensitive skin of the perineum. For those people lucky enough to have a well-maintained private pool, they can do some extremely gentle aquatic exercise once they have healed, shortly after the birth, as bathing is not contraindicated. However, if you have access to a pool and want to start exercising before six weeks, it is courteous to get medical approval.

Normally, exercise after caesarean sections is delayed beyond six weeks but, providing the surgeon approves, there are no contraindications to starting aquatic exercise sooner. After all, postoperative patients often have hydrotherapy.

Physiological Adaptations After Childbirth

All the changes to the pregnant body gradually revert to the pre-pregnant state. However, relaxin remains in the body for about five months, and ligaments, and therefore joints, are vulnerable for that time. Dynamic full range joint work should therefore not be done until five months after giving birth.

All the beneficial 'training' effects which happened to the cardiovascular system during pregnancy gradually disappear, in the same way that all the beneficial effects of training vanish once the training has ceased. In fact, if training is started shortly after giving birth, then peak performance may well develop. Several elite women athletes have achieved their personal best shortly after giving birth. For the normal woman, though, the last thing they feel like is undertaking serious athletic training. Often women feel exhausted in the first months after childbirth, probably through having disturbed nights and fraught days. It can come as a shock that such a tiny person can take up so much time and need so much attention! If the baby is a sibling for another child, then it is even more tiring for the mother,

as they have to see to the needs of the rest of the family. The hormonal adjustments may also add to the feeling of tiredness. In some ways, women are better motivated to exercise after the birth than before, as they want to return their figures to pre-pregnant states. However, sheer tiredness may make this impossible. On the other hand, if inertia can be overcome, participation in a properly conducted exercise session can be positively energizing.

Structure and Aims of a Postnatal Aquatic Exercise

The aims of exercise are to help the body return to its prenatal state. This means strengthening the damaged muscles, the pelvic floor and the abdominals (see below for details) and, by aerobic training, trying to maintain the enhanced aerobic performance gained during pregnancy. It is also important for the new mother to have some enjoyment and some time that is 'just for her'. The babies seem to appreciate this, as evidenced by the line of babies at the pool-side, asleep in their travel chairs. Perhaps it is the warm atmosphere, or the music, but by their calmness, the babies give the impression of approving of their mother's exercising.

As regards the format of the Aquarobics session, this should be similar to a normal but gentle class for young women. It should be a total body work-out, lasting 30 to 45 minutes and be enjoyable, physically beneficial, innervating and concentrate for some of the time in facilitating the changes from pregnancy to the non-pregnant state, as seen below.

RESTORATION OF NORMAL POSTURE

It is important to re-educate normal posture, and when the mothers realize that pulling in their abdomen can also help them to look better, they are cooperative. The body needs to be correctly aligned, so that the head is over the shoulders, the spine is erect, there are normal spinal curves (not exaggerated), the hips and knees are straight and the body weight falls just in front of the ankle joint.

ABDOMINAL MUSCLE RE-EDUCATION

Posture will be helped when the abdominal muscles start to return to normal. When pregnant, the vertical abdominal muscles (the recti abdomini) separate to make more space for the baby, and this gap can be clearly felt for some time after the birth. If they are worked too hard when the gap is still present, the muscles will 'dome'. These muscles must not be worked until the gap has virtually gone. It is thought by some that working the oblique muscles, by doing twisting exercises, can increase the gap in the recti, so such exercises should be avoided until the gap has gone. Pulling the abdomen in as much as pos-

sible works the transversus, but it will also help the 'gap' to mend. It is better to assess the size of the gap between the recti out of the water. The mothers lie on their backs with knees bent and feet on the floor. They are instructed to do a pelvic tilt (flatten their spine on to the floor), then raise their heads, and possibly the shoulders, by sliding the hands up towards the knees. If the abdominal muscles 'dome' outwards down the midline the two recti muscles are still separate. The gap can be felt by palpating in the midline. As soon as the gap has gone and there is no bulging on a gentle abdominal curl, then the abdominal exercises in Section IV, page 153, can be started.

BREAST CARE

Women who are breastfeeding should try to feed the baby shortly before exercising. One result of poor posture when feeding (either breast or bottle) is pain around the neck and shoulders. Advise on correct seated posture when feeding,

Table 7.4
Summary of objectives of postnatal exercise

Aims	Means
1. To facilitate the body's return to the prenatal state	To strengthen weakened muscles, the pelvic floor and abdominals
2. To enhance cardiovascular fitness	Gentle aerobic training
3. To correct posture	Improve alignment and tone postural muscles
4. To enhance well-being	By participating in structured general exercise
5. To provide an opportunity for relaxation	Floating and generally having fun!
6. To provide an opportunity for social support, and a potential pathway for professional advice	By arranging a communal rest period afterwards

perhaps using a pillow under the baby to avoid stooping, could resolve the problem. In terms of exercise, some upper body strengthening and gentle mobility work may counteract this discomfort. It is very important to wear a bra that is truly supportive; nursing bras do not always conform to this requirement.

PELVIC FLOOR

Returning the stretched and damaged pelvic floor to its prenatal function is probably the most important aspect to postnatal exercise. It is important that this is correctly taught. Ideally the muscles of the pelvic floor should be able to contract alone, without linking their contraction with strong ones of the abdominal muscles, gluteals or hip adductors — all of which should remain largely at rest.

The most effective imagery is to imagine having diarrhoea whilst on the M1, 5 miles short of the next service station. Squeeze the back passage as though trying to hold on. Next bring the contraction slightly forward, as though trying to stop the flow of urine. The final stage is to be able to contract the internal muscles of the vagina, and the best way to check whether this is happening is by using 'natural bio-feedback' at home — either by inserting a finger in the vagina and feeling the squeeze, or during intercourse when the partner can confirm whether or not there is a muscle contraction.

Once a pelvic floor contraction is mastered, it should be practised so as to work both the aerobic and the power fibres of the pelvic floor muscles. To work the former, tighten and hold the contraction for 4 seconds. Repeat only once or twice. To work the power fibres, go for a maximum contraction, but only hold it for 1 second. Repeat four or five times. Breathing should be normal throughout.

Appendix 7.1

AMERICAN COLLEGE OF OBSTETRICS AND GYNECOLOGY GUIDELINES FOR EXERCISE IN PREGNANCY

The following guidelines refer to dry-land exercise. they do not take account of the lower heart rate when immersed. It is now evident that antenatal exercise needs to be gentle, comfortable and enjoyable.

1. Maternal HR should not exceed 140 beats/minute.
2. Strenuous activities should not exceed 15 min duration.
3. No exercises should be performed in the supine position after the fourth month of gestation is completed.
4. Exercises that employ the Valsalva manoeuvre should be avoided.
5. Calorific intake should be adequate to meet not only the extra energy needs of pregnancy, but also of the exercise performed.
6. Maternal core temperature should not exceed 38.5 °C.

SUGGESTED GUIDELINE FOR AQUATIC EXERCISE

Maternal heart rate should not exceed 130 beats/minute and this intensity of exercise should not be maintained for more than 20 minutes.

References

American College of Obstetrics and Gynecology (1994) *Exercise During Pregnancy and The Post-partum Period.* ACOG Technical Bulletin 189. ACOG, Washington, DC.

Berry MJ, McMurray RG and Katz VL (1989) Pulmonary and ventilatory responses to pregnancy, immersion and exercise. *J Appl Physiol* 66(2): 857–862.

Cugell DW, Frank NR, Gaensler EA and Badger TL (1953) Pulmonary function in pregnancy: I Serial observation in normal women. *Am Rev Tuberc Pulm Dis* **67**: 568–597.

Gee JB, Packer LBS, Millen JER and Robin ED (1967) Pulmonary mechanics during pregnancy. *J Clinic Invest* **46**: 945–952.

Katz VL (1991) Physiologic changes during normal pregnancy. *Curr Opin Obstet Gynecol* 3(6): 750–758.

Knuttgen HG and Emerson K (1974) Physiological response to pregnancy at rest and during exercise. *J Appl Physiol* **36**: 549–553.

McMurray RG and Katz VL (1990) Thermoregulation in pregnancy. Implications for exercise. *Sport Med* **10**(3): 146–158.

Sternfeld B (1997) Physical activity and pregnancy outcome. Review and recommendations. *Sport Med* **23**(1): 33–47.

Wallace AM and Engstron JL (1987) The effects of aerobic exercise on the pregnant woman, fetus and pregnancy outcome: a review. *J Nurse Midwifery* **32**(5): 277–290.

Wallace AM, Boyer DB, Dan A and Holm K (1986) Aerobic exercise, maternal self-esteem, and physical discomforts during pregnancy. *J Nurse Midwifery* **31**(6): 255–262.

Zeanah M and Schlosser SP (1993) The adherence to ACOG guidelines on exercise during pregnancy: effect on pregnancy outcome. *J Obs Gynecol Neonatal Nursing* **22**(4): 329–335.

8

Inflammatory and Degenerative Arthropathies

The group of people who are the most appreciative of aquatherapy, in my experience, are those who suffer from arthritis. For such people, whose normal, everyday activities may cause considerable pain, the ability (when immersed) to perform simple, normal movements without discomfort is a source of great joy and physical freedom. These statements are gross generalizations, as there are many kinds of arthritis and a wide spectrum of pain and disability within each clinical group. There is also the possibility that inappropriate exercise can make the underlying condition worse, so it is important that any professional responsible for conducting aquatic exercise not only understands the underlying condition and the degree of disease activity, but is able to assess the needs of that particular client on that particular day.

This chapter will attempt to provide some background knowledge on all except the very rare arthritic conditions and, in each case, point out any factors which have practical implications about the way in which the exercise is carried out. Because physiotherapists should already have a good knowledge of the various conditions, they may want to go directly to the accompanying practical implications. On the other hand, the disease descriptions may be helpful revision for student physiotherapists.

What is Arthropathy?

Arthro means joint, and *pathy* means disease. An arthropathy is therefore a 'sick' joint. '*Itis*' means inflammation. Arthritis should therefore literally mean an inflammation of a joint, but this term can be a misnomer because joints are not always inflamed in all types of arthritis. Whereas arthropathy might be a more specific medical term, the accepted lay description for this group of diseases is arthritis.

Generally speaking, the arthropathies can be divided into two types – mechanical and inflammatory. Whereas the former can sometimes affect only one joint, and may have been precipitated by a previous injury, inflammatory joint disease may not only damage joints throughout the whole body, but is sometimes associated with damage to totally different systems, such as the digestive system or the kidneys. However, such generalized classification is an over-simplification of the true spectrum of disease. There are almost as many varieties of arthropathy as there are joints in the body (180). Nevertheless, the number of people who suffer from mechanical arthritis (otherwise known as degenerative or osteoarthritis [OA]) is probably greater than the sum of all those with the other rarer forms of joint disease put together.

These other arthritic diseases, which fall broadly into the category of 'inflammatory', can be further subdivided into those of autoimmune origin (e.g. rheumatoid arthritis [RA]) or ankylosing spondylitis [AS]), those of infective origin (e.g. bacterial arthritis), those of general metabolic dysfunction (e.g. gout) and those which do not fit into any of the other categories, but which are systemic and therefore involve damage to differing tissues and systems in the body. The knowledge gained and the resultant technological developments of recent years has cast new lights on some of these distressing, painful and sometimes life-threatening conditions. It is to be hoped that further research will lead to a full understanding of the cellular, physiological and genetic factors so that the underlying cause will be known. Only then will there be a more effective treatment for those already suffering, and perhaps even total prevention and eradication of the diseases.

Disease Stages: Acute or Chronic

Before launching into specific pathologies, there are some general points which have implications for all sufferers of arthritic conditions. The first concerns the status of affected joints, whether they are acute or chronic. Also to be considered are the temperature and depth of the water when exercising and the accessibility of the pool building and the pool itself. Whatever the diagnosis of an arthropathy, the terms *acute* and *chronic* are used to describe the severity of disease in joints. The classic signs of an *acute* joint are redness, warmth and swelling. Any attempt to move such a joint will produce immediate pain, and a prob-

able increase in the protective muscle spasm. Such spasms are not necessarily bad as they could be looked on as nature's way of providing splinting to prevent movement. A *chronic* inflamed joint is one in which the acute inflammatory process has minimized or resolved, but in which damage will have occurred to all or some of the structures within and around it. Between the two states of acute and chronic there is an intermediary category known as *subacute*.

The treatment of all acute conditions is rest, and aquatic exercise is therefore likely to be inappropriate at this time. An exception might be for an individual who has one or two acute joints but where the others are subacute or chronic. If the acute joint can be immobilized in some way, then the advantages of immersion on the remainder of the body may outweigh the risk of an exacerbation in that one joint. Aquatic therapy may be given to such individuals, but the management in such cases is highly specialized and needs not only approval from the rheumatologist concerned, but requires the skills of a physiotherapist and the facilities of a hydrotherapy pool.

Aquatic therapy is most beneficial for those whose arthropathy is chronic or quiescent. It is not only extremely therapeutic to damaged joints by facilitating mobility, strengthening weakened musculature and permitting the pain-free practice of functional manoeuvres such as walking, but it is possibly the only way that general exercise can be carried out painlessly and enjoyably. Furthermore, the increased cardiovascular activity that comes with exercise enhances well-being and may release endorphins. Hall (1993) compared β-endorphin levels in rheumatoid arthritis (RA) patients resting during immersion with exercise during immersion, all in thermoneutral water. Against expectations, she found that β-endorphin levels were reduced in both groups when

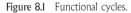

Figure 8.1 Functional cycles.

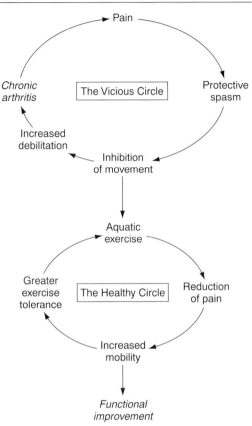

Figure 8.2 Illustration of synovial joint.

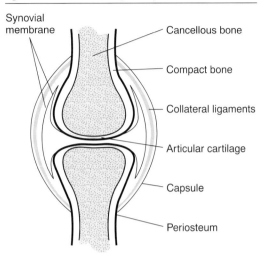

edge of normal joint anatomy in order to appreciate the abnormalities that accompany the disease process. All physiotherapists will have such detailed knowledge, but the aquatic exercise coaches will not normally have studied anatomy in as much depth. Figure 8.2 shows a synovial joint and Table 8.1 is a revision of the different specialist tissues that make up the complicated set of interfaces which constitutes a synovial joint.

Factors Affecting Aquatic Therapy for Arthropathies

Temperature

A characteristic of many of the arthritic conditions listed below, is that pain is made worse when cold, and reduced when warm. This refers to the body as a whole, as well as to any affected, individual joint. (An exception to this is when one or more joints are undergoing an acute inflammatory reaction, in which case they will be hot and swollen and may benefit from being cooled down.) The average swimming pool is kept at a

compared with the control. She postulates that this effect (which was not significant) is the result of the haemodilution and other physiological adaptations caused by immersion.

Figure 8.1 shows that the usual vicious circle associated with joint disease, of pain, spasm, inhibition of movement, and general debility, can be broken, leading to a positive outcome that maximizes function and well-being and minimizes pain.

Revision of Joint Anatomy

In order to break the vicious circle and maximize the positive, it is vital that all professionals who work with arthritis sufferers have a good knowl-

Table 8.1
Different tissues found in and around synovial joints

Tissue	Function
Bone	Bone is specialized connective tissue impregnated with mineral salts. The outer part of bone ends are made of ivory-like compact bone, to provide strength and support. Bone is continually being remoulded and restructured.
Articular or hyaline cartilage	The extremely dense, hard, smooth 'cap' to that part of a bone which comes into direct contact with other similar surfaces. Designed to minimize friction. Hard wearing, but prone to degenerative change. In adults it has no blood supply.
Synovial membrane	The delicate 'nasal-type' membrane which lines all other structures within the joint that are not covered in articular cartilage. Main function is to secrete synovial fluid.
Synovial fluid	Has two vital roles. 1. It is similar to engine oil in that it lubricates the moving parts thereby minimizing friction. 2. It acts as a supply system to adjoining tissues, especially articular cartilage, providing nutrients and oxygen and removing waste products.
Intra-articular structures	For example, intravertebral discs in the spine and menisci in knees and wrist. These are very hard wearing, made of fibrocartilage and are there to dissipate the forces, and transmit load, by acting somewhat like a washer. They are prone to traumatic damage and degenerative changes.
Capsule	A specialized envelope that delineates and encapsulates the joint. Made of strong, inelastic collagen. It binds the bones together and gives some stability.
Ligaments	Composed, like the capsule, of dense masses of collagen fibres, but arranged in strong bands (e.g. the medial ligament of the knee), or in other places requiring stability. Ligaments join bone to bone.
Blood	Blood is a liquid connective tissue, which acts as the main transport system of the body. All tissues require oxygen and nutrients and the removal of the waste products of metabolism. Blood carries them to the appropriate part of the body for further processing or removal. It also carries the chemical messengers that act as the switches for metabolism. All the tissues around joints require a good blood supply, apart from articular cartilage in adults.
Nerve	Joints require a rich supply of nerves to control the complicated process of movement. Nerve endings in the capsule and ligaments are mechanoreceptors, which register movement, proprioceptors which register the position of the joint and specialized nerve endings, nocioceptors, which register pain. Blood supply is controlled by sympathetic nerves.
Muscles	Muscles are the engines of the musculoskeletal system. A muscle consists of specialized muscle fibres which have the ability to contract and be stretched. One end of the muscle is connected to the bone by a strong collagen tendon and the other end by some form of connective tissue anchor. Muscles are arranged in groups and work together as agonist and antagonist.* They pass over at least one joint and adapt their length to bring about the required movement or control unwanted movement. They have to keep the body upright against gravity. They are composed of specialist fibres which have their own nerve control. They respond to work by getting larger (training), and to inactivity or pain by wasting away.

* See Glossary

temperature considerably below that of a hydrotherapy pool, and this has practical implications for aquatic exercise for people with arthropathy. Generally speaking, people with joint disease far prefer the warmer temperature of a thermoneutral (see Glossary) hydrotherapy pool, although the excessive temperature of some hydrotherapy pools (i.e. above 34 °C) whilst being pleasant for the arthritic joints, can be debilitating. An ideal temperature for exercising with chronic arthritis would be thermoneutral, but it is very difficult to achieve this outside a hospital environment. Nonetheless, correct teaching, and keeping the most of the body submerged, means that aquatic exercise for people with arthritis can be carried out in most swimming pools. Whereas, in the UK, it is not recommended that such activity takes place if the water is less than 27 °C, in the United States, pool water is generally kept lower than that, at about 24 °C. Furthermore YMCA classes for people with arthritis are taking place in many hundreds of pools around the United States, and are generally held to be helpful. So perhaps the pool temperature is not as critical an issue as conventionally believed?

Accessibility to the Pool

Whereas all hospital hydrotherapy pools are designed with good access for the disabled in mind, this is not necessarily true for swimming pools. Often there is a long walk from the changing area to the pool itself, and this may prevent those with feet and leg disabilities from reaching the water. Pool floors tend to be of non-slip ceramic tiles, and this surface can be particularly painful to walk on. Clients should be encouraged to wear slippers or shoes between the changing rooms and the pool-side.

Entry into the water can also be difficult. Most arthritis sufferers would find a ladder impossible to

negotiate and will require easy access steps with handrails both sides. Legislation in many countries, including the UK, now makes easy access for those with disability compulsory; despite the law, however, it does not always happen.

Mechanical Arthritis (osteoarthritis)

Osteoarthritis (OA) is also known as degenerative arthritis, degenerative joint disease, arthritis deformans and 'wear-and-tear' arthritis. It is the commonest form of arthritis, a chronic degenerative disease of joints with exacerbations of acute inflammation. These acute episodes are not as severe or consistent as in many of the other forms of arthritis. As its alternative names imply, it is primarily mechanical and degenerative in origin. It is found all over the world and was known in ancient times, as demonstrated by typical OA changes to stone-age skeletons. It is primarily a condition of older people, and is sometimes looked upon as an exacerbation of the wear-and-tear changes that can happen in certain joints with age.

OA can be a disease of just one joint, and in this case is often thought to be the result of previous trauma to that joint, or some mechanical malalignment which eventually precipitates the degenerative changes. The trauma may have been mild, and have happened a long time ago, but, rather like the effect of a grain of sand among ball-bearings, it may lead to an inexorable accumulation of damage. OA can also be a disease of many joints, and this may involve some genetic predisposition. There is a sex difference in the distribution of affected joints, the order of incidence for men being most commonly the hip, then the knee, spine, ankle, shoulder and fingers. For women the commonest joint to be affected is the knee, followed, in order, by finger, spine, hip, ankle and shoulder (Thomson *et al.*, 1991). (This difference may be biological, or reflect conventional lifestyles.) As well as trauma being a causative factor, OA can also arise as a result of other diseases or infections.

Typical Changes

There is erosion of articular cartilage and a breakdown of collagen. The cartilage softens, flakes and eventually can be virtually destroyed, especially centrally over the weight-bearing area. At the edges there is a thickening of the articular cartilage. All of this means that there will no longer be a smooth joint surface, and friction will be increased. Once the articular cartilage is no longer there to protect the bone, that becomes cystic (see Glossary) and damaged. Osteophytes (resembling miniature bony stalactites) form at the edges of the bone, and further impede movement. Occasionally these, or loose bits of cartilage, can break off and become jammed between the bone ends, causing the joint to become 'locked'.

The synovial membrane becomes thickened and, as part of the inflammatory process, produces too much synovial fluid in much the same way that the nasal membranes produce surplus fluid in a cold. This leads to swelling. Initially this may be quite sudden and dramatic, as in a 'housemaid's knee'. Eventually the whole joint becomes enlarged and the range of movement is severely restricted and painful. All the tissues around the joint degenerate, including the fabric of the capsule and the ligaments, and the joint may develop a posture which eventually leads to a typical deformity. The muscles that act on that joint get weaker, partly as a reflex response to damage, and partly through disuse. As the joint cannot move through the whole range, the muscles are denied the opportunity to work through their normal range, and they atrophy (see Glossary) as a result.

OA does not spread from one joint to another as a disease or an infection would. However, because it can be caused by mechanical malalignment, a dysfunction of one joint (e.g. the right hip) may cause a limp, which could eventually cause mechanical damage to either knee, the other hip or the lumbar spine, depending on which other joints are taking the strain of the affected ones. Given that the individual may have a genetic predisposition to developing OA, as

---

Table 8.2
Implications for aquatic exercise in OA

Aims	Potential hazards
To encourage normal functional movement patterns, especially walking	Providing that the Aquarobics principles are observed — none!
To take damaged joints through as full a range of movement as possible	
To strengthen all muscles acting on the affected joints, those in the surrounding region and functional muscles such as the abdominals	
To improve aerobic fitness	
To release endorphins and reduce pain	

manifested by the original joint, then it is easy to understand how other joints can become affected.

The maxim 'use it or lose it' is the best way of retarding these degenerative changes, and aquatic exercise is a good way of 'using it'. By trying to maintain mechanically correct movement and working the muscles against resistance, the degenerative process can be slowed down. In fact, as many more people show signs of OA when X-rayed than actually have any symptoms, it is probably possible to reverse some of the changes.

Inflammatory Arthritis

There are very many diseases that fall into this category – but many of them are extremely rare. A general characteristic of most is localized joint pain and accompanying systemic fatigue. Although the precise aetiology (see Glossary) of the majority of inflammatory arthropathies is unknown, many are thought to be autoimmune and multisystem in origin, and it could be that the immune system plays an important role in feelings of fatigue. Advice by rheumatologists is to try to avoid excessive fatigue, and this has inevitable consequences for exercise. Probably aquatic exercise is less tiring than weight-bearing exercise, but it can still have adverse reactions. Such reactions may be precipitated if the temperature of the water is too warm or too cold.

What is an Autoimmune Disease?

The term 'autoimmune' disease (i.e. a condition where the immune system attacks self tissues as though they were foreign cells to be eliminated), is one that is frequently associated with inflammatory arthritis, as well as with a number of other distressing conditions, such as 'juvenile diabetes' and multiple sclerosis. It is not that uncommon for totally different autoimmune syndromes to be present in the same individual. Recent research into immunology has produced a broad theory of the underlying mechanism of autoimmune diseases and the fact that they can coexist is perfectly logical.

In order to develop an autoimmune disease, any individual must usually have a certain genetic predisposition in terms of their tissue-typing characteristics (technically their human leukocyte antigen [HLA] haplotype). The extent to which there is inherited predisposition (or indeed protection) varies between autoimmune diseases, but even those most tightly linked to HLA haplotype are not strictly hereditary diseases, as shown by studies with inherited twins. Clearly there are environmental factors that come into play as well. As an example, there is virtually no risk of contacting ankylosing spondylitis (AS) unless a person is of the tissue type designated HLA-B27. However, although B27 is an unambiguous risk factor for AS (and, indeed, for a variety of other autoimmune diseases), only a fraction of the people bearing that antigen will actually get the disease. Similar considerations apply to RA, although here the genetics of susceptibility, in terms of tissue typing, is rather more complex.

A generally accepted model of how autoimmunity occurs is that it involves 'molecular mimicry'. Immune cells activated by a particular protein fragment of an infectious agent mount an attack on protein fragments of self-tissue, parts of which (by chance) are similar to part of the microbe. In other words, the immune cells are 'fooled' into thinking that they are still rejecting the infection, and therefore attempt to destroy a part of 'self'. How this mimicry concept accounts for HLA association with particular diseases is the basis of a number of hypotheses, the most recent being the 'three-way mimicry theory' (Baum, 1997), details of which are beyond the scope of this book. Suffice to say that modern cell biology is close to explaining the molecular basis of the autoimmune arthropathies such as AS and RA.

Rheumatoid Arthritis

Rheumatoid arthritis (RA) is the commonest of these diseases, and is found all over the world. It is a generalized disease of connective tissue, and therefore affects joints as well as other systems. The sex ratio is approximately three women to one male. It can occur at any age above 16, but the onset is most commonly during the thirties and forties. The prevalence is about 37 per thousand population (Berry, 1983).

It usually first appears suddenly as polyarthritis (see Glossary), causing pain and swelling in several of the joints of the hands and feet. Generally speaking it starts in the periphery, the MTP joints in the feet and the PIP and MCP joints of the hands (see Glossary), and then moves centrally, attacking the subtalar, ankles, knees and sometimes hips in the lower extremities, and the carpal joints, wrists, elbows, shoulders, upper cervical spine and temperomandibular joints. Fortunately, not all joints are acutely inflamed at the same time, but the joints can eventually become destroyed.

The nature of the disease is unpredictable, as it can completely disappear after affecting only one or two joints. In the worst (fortunately rare) scenario, it can be an extremely painful, crippling and deforming disease accompanied by generalized fatigue, but with accompanying vasculitis, cardiac or respiratory complications or other systemic manifestations. The damage to the joints can be quite profound. Initially, the synovial membrane is inflamed and the subsequent immune response causes thickening and proliferation. The joint cartilage becomes damaged, and the bone can become cystic. The erosion of subchondral bone leads to the development of typical deformities and can cause subluxation. Blood vessels are affected throughout the body and the spleen can become enlarged.

The disease process can stop at any time, but may leave behind a residue of mechanically damaged joints, which are then prone to further mechanical OA insult. On the other hand, a few fortunate sufferers only have short-lived problems with one or two joints, which can resolve, leaving no damage whatsoever.

Treatment in the acute stage is rest, and there are a battery of specific pharmaceutical agents available to minimize inflammation and control the pain and the disease process. The end-line drug for many people is steroids, and long-term steroid use causes osteoporosis. The possibility of subluxation of the atlanto-occipital joint (see Glossary) (which is fatal), and of osteoporotic collapse, must be remembered during all forms of physical therapy.

Special Considerations for Aquatic Exercise for RA Sufferers

1. The water should be chest-high and preferably at a temperature of 32–34 °C. If any joints are acutely inflamed then medical approval should have been received beforehand. If only one joint (e.g. a wrist) is acute, then it may be possible to wear an immersible, non-buoyant, wrist splint, so that the rest of the body can be exercised without risk of damage to the vulnerable area.

2. As the feet as likely to have been damaged by RA, walking on textured tiled surfaces is likely

to be extremely uncomfortable. Participants should therefore be advised to wear shoes or slippers right up to the place of immersion. If this is a swimming pool, then special arrangements may need to be made with the management. Alternatively, appropriate footwear can be worn in the water. There are specially designed water immersible trainers available, designed for aquatic coaches. However, the rheumatoid deformities, which often make the foot wider, may exclude the use of these. If nothing else, thick socks can be worn getting to, and even into, the water.

3. The joints of the fingers, carpus and wrist will probably have been damaged. Any pressure on these joints is extremely painful. It is better to avoid hand-holding, especially by other clients who may have different arthritic conditions and therefore be unaware of the potential for pain caused by the inadvertent 'squeeze' of a handshake. It may be painful to hold on to equipment such as floats, but woggles are probably comfortable as the whole hand can go around them, rather like holding a walking frame or a bannister.

4. If the neck has been affected by RA, then lying supine, with or without floats, could be potentially very dangerous. Subluxation of the atlanto-occipital joint is a rare complication of RA. If this joint does happen, then the damage to the spinal cord is probably terminal. It is therefore suggested that RA sufferers who have ever had upper cervical pain should not be asked to lie on their backs during an aquatic exercise session, unless the session is conducted by a therapist who not only knows how to apply support to the head and neck in a totally safe manner, but knows when it would be too risky so to do.

5. Extra time is needed for dressing and undressing, and help may be required. In a swimming pool changing room, the seats tend to be too low. If there are no dedicated facilities for disabled people then it may be necessary to arrange for a higher chair and a lavatory with easy access for the disabled.

6. As fatigue is a concomitant of RA, it is better to have short sessions, at least initially. The warmer water, necessary because it is more comfortable to RA joints, is more tiring than cooler water. Participants should be advised not to rush home immediately after the session, but to sit down and have a drink and a rest.

7. If the session is dedicated to people with arthritis, then it is helpful to timetable such a rest in a social setting. Water is a natural leveller, and it often opens the verbal floodgates. Sometimes arthritis sufferers do not have the same opportunities to meet with friends and go out to places of entertainment because of difficulties with access. This can lead to social isolation which can, for a few people, become as serious a problem as the RA. Participation in aquatic sessions, and having an opportunity afterwards to talk to fellow sufferers who become friends, helps with the realization that they are not alone with their problems.

8. As morning stiffness, which can last from five minutes to three hours, is one of the commonest symptoms of RA, it is better to hold therapy sessions in the afternoon or early evening.

Session Content

I asked an RA sufferer who had been attending my clinic intermittently for about 20 years, for hydrotherapy, what it was that kept her coming. Her reply was, 'It's like all my elastic bands have been loosened.' Her description of RA was a feeling that her body consisted of stretched elastic bands. Gentle exercise in the water released the tension in those bands and provided her with additional mobility.

Obviously, the opportunity to move through as large a normal range of movement as possible, in a supported pain-free environment, is immensely beneficial, and exercises to maintain and increase mobility are therefore an important aim of therapy. It is also important to maintain muscle strength as, without exercise, there is muscle atrophy. If the physical limitations allow for large-scale movements to be performed so that there is a rise in heart rate, then there will be some aerobic training, and this may lead to the release of endorphins.

The traditional treatment for RA was rest, as it was felt that exercise could cause exacerbations of the joint disease. This belief was questioned by several studies initiated in Scandinavia. Lyngberg and colleagues (1988) found that sufferers of RA were initially 'unfit' when assessed by various fitness parameters including VO_2 and quadriceps strength, but improved in many ways by participating in a training programme. It was found that the beneficial results were enhanced if the training took place in water (Danneskiold et al., 1987).

Two more recent studies (Hall, 1993; Baum, 1994) also found certain benefits from Aquarobics-type exercises in warm water. These benefits were subjective, however, and not of statistical significance.

Because weight-bearing through affected joints is painful, water may be the only medium that allows exercise of sufficient intensity to bring about the desired cardiovascular and well-being effects. Perhaps the sufferer will start their aquatic exercise in the warm water of a hydrotherapy pool, in the form of specific rehabilitation exercises. Even in a small hydrotherapy pool one can exercise all four limbs at once sufficiently vigorously to get breathless. By doing this, rather than carrying out isolated exercises for just one limb

at a time, the effort will improve cardiovascular function, enhance well-being and probably also be more effective than just the original strengthening and flexibility programme. It is hoped that they will then be able to continue classes in their neighbourhood swimming pool, and that this will maintain and improve not only specific joint and muscle function, but also help them to feel fitter and less tired generally.

The objectives of such an aquatic session will be to improve functional ability, particularly walking, to mobilize joints, to strengthen muscles, to enhance overall fitness and, most importantly, to provide pleasure. It is easier to achieve these objectives if the depth of the water is between waist and chest height.

Juvenile Arthritis

This is an acute form of arthritis that affects children. There are different syndromes within the general description of juvenile arthritis (JA) with differing prognoses. One form of the disease, which affects children commonly under the age of 5, is an acute-onset illness, with a rash, spiky fever and enlarged lymph nodes, liver and spleen. There may be pericarditis or pleurisy and the child can be very ill. The symptoms usually remit when in their teens, but there may well be permanent joint damage. Another form of JA that comes at any age has only joint involvement, usually affecting a number of joints, without the systemic features. Another form has only a few joints affected initially, but others may subsequently become involved (Berry, 1983; Ansell, 1991).

Children with JA require the intervention of a team of differing professionals to help them to lead as normal a life as possible, at home, at school and socially. Hydrotherapy is helpful throughout, but in the early stages treatment will be very gentle. The aim then is to reduce pain, to do gentle mobility work, which is often more comfortable in the water, thereby helping to prevent deformities developing. As the joints settle down, then more active therapy aimed at rehabilitating walking, regaining strength and mobility can be commenced, often on a one-to-one basis. As soon as possible, active group work is started, and this is more likely to continue within the confines of a specialist unit under the care of a paediatric hydrotherapist.

Once the active phase of the disease is over, and the child becomes an adult, aquatic keep fit classes may be the easiest form of exercise. Such classes will help to maintain independence and may enhance cardiovascular fitness. Most importantly, though, they provide an opportunity for leisure, relaxation and enjoyment in a normal environment.

The aims of treatment for adults who had JA will be the same as for those people with RA; namely to reduce pain, to prevent deformities, to increase muscle strength and joint mobility and to maintain independence. The same precautions will apply.

Ankylosing Spondylitis

Ankylosing spondylitis (AS) is an autoimmune disease that affects men more than women, in the ratio of 2.4:1 (NASS, 1997). The onset is usually between the ages of 15 and 40. About 6 people per 1000 suffer from AS, but it is a condition which is thought often to be misdiagnosed. As with all autoimmune diseases, tissue typing is important, and 96% of patients fall into the category of HLA B27-positive. (Because there is a genetic predisposition, the disease is 30 times more common among family members than in the general population. It is characterized by periods of acute exacerbations and long periods of quiescence.)

A characteristic sign of AS is being woken by acute pain and suffering stiffness for some time after rising, especially in the early stages of the disease. The first joints to be affected are often the sacroiliac joints, with a synovitis and, from there, the disease spreads up the spine and to the rib joints. If severe, it can involve the hips and shoulder joints. Periosteum, ligaments and muscle junctions become infiltrated and new bone proliferates, and the tissues around the joints become infiltrated with bone, so that movement can eventually become impossible. If the thorax and ribs are affected, then breathing will be restricted.

The characteristic deformity is a fixed spinal flexion, and this is very disabling. Exercises are essential to try to maintain mobility and prevent deformity. Hydrotherapy is useful, but probably not sufficient on its own to limit deformity. Sufferers need to embark on a daily flexibility and extensor strengthening exercise routine.

The Aims of Aquatic Therapy

1. It is necessary to mobilize the affected joints, to try to prevent new bone formation from ankylosing them. As far as the spine is concerned, this primarily means extension in order to counteract the deformity which causes flexion.

2. Exercises need to encourage ventilation, to keep the rib cage mobile, and this means getting breathless. A byproduct of such exercise may be improved cardiovascular fitness. Some severe AS sufferers may already have restricted pulmonary function because of the disease process, and it must be remembered that

hydrostatic pressure can put additional strain on breathing. It may therefore be necessary, at least initially, to be in waist-high water. However, as soon as possible, shoulder-high water should be used, to immerse the damaged thoracic spine. Always, the emphasis needs to be on exercises that extend, rather than flex, the spine. Spinal rotation and side flexion are also important. Hips and shoulders can be put through exercises in all possible planes of movement.

Systemic Lupus Erythematosus

This once extremely rare disease is becoming more common, or better diagnosed. It is another autoimmune disease, affecting women to men in the ratio of 9:1. The onset is during the child-bearing years. The name originates from the butterfly rash, sometimes found on the face, which used to be thought of as wolf-like (lupus). The symptoms are very variable, but may include joint involvement, similar to that in RA, but usually symmetrical whereas RA may be asymmetrical. As the joint involvement is non-erosive, the prognosis is better than in RA. There is often associated systemic disease, of the kidneys, the cardiovascular system, the gastrointestinal system or the central nervous system perhaps causing depression, all of which is potentially more serious and disabling than the intermittent joint disease. SLE is prone to episodes of exacerbations and remissions and may remit altogether.

IMPLICATIONS FOR AQUATIC THERAPY

There are no particular implications for aquatic exercise for SLE sufferers, apart from the fact that fatigue should be avoided. This is probably more important than in other arthritic conditions because the disease affects so many of the body systems. It is therefore better to start very gently and build up the tolerance to exercise, observing the Aquarobics principle of 'sensible moderation'.

Polymyalgia Rheumatica

Only older people are affected by this unpleasant condition. The classic symptoms are early morning pain and stiffness, often around the shoulders, of such severity that it can take several hours to loosen up sufficiently to get dressed. It is accompanied by fatigue and can have serious complications if untreated. It is easily mistaken for degenerative arthritis or cervical spondylitis but, unlike the other two conditions, can be totally resolved with a low dose of steroids. Although this condition may be more prevalent in the unfit elderly, it is possible that it may affect an aquatic exercise enthusiast. Aquatic teachers should therefore be aware that if there is an unexpected onset of pain and stiffness in older people, usually around the shoulders, but possibly in the buttocks, they should be directed to their doctor.

Metabolic or Crystal Arthropathy

There are several forms of metabolic diseases which cause joint pain and dysfunction. Of these the commonest, by far, is gout.

Gout

Gout is a disorder of protein metabolism that results in an inability to excrete uric acid. The result is a build-up crystals of sodium urate, which are then carried around in blood vessels and eventually form deposits in various classical sites. Historically, this was mainly thought to be the metatarsal-phalangeal joint of the first toe, but it is now known that crystals can be deposited anywhere, but they tend to be peripheral. If this happens, there is an acute, extremely painful inflammation, which cannot be exercised. Gout is, fortunately, controllable by drugs (allopurinol and colchicine). It should therefore not present as a problem in hydrotherapy or aquatic therapy.

References

Ansell BM, Rudges S and Schaller JG (eds) (1992) *Colour Atlas of Paediatric Rheumatology*. Wolfe, Aylesbury.

Baum G (1994) The effect of Aquarobics on mobility in chronic rheumatoid arthritis. Unpublished MSc Thesis. Manchester Metropolitan University.

Baum H (1997) Molecular mimicry with MHC-derived peptides: does this underlie MHC association with autoimmune disease? *Biochem Soc Trans* **25**: 636–642.

Berry H (1983) Rheumatoid arthritis. In: *Rheumatology and Rehabilitation* (eds Berry H, Hamilton E and Goodwill J), Croom Helm, London.

Danneskiold-Samsoe B, Lyngberg K, Risum T and Telling M (1987) The effect of water exercise therapy given to patients with RA. *Scand J Rehab Med* **19**(1): 31–35.

Hall J (1993) The therapeutic and physiological effects of hydrotherapy on patients with rheumatoid arthritis. MPhil Thesis. University of Bath.

Lyngberg K, Danneskiold-Samsoe B and Halskov O (1988) The effect of physical training on patients with rheumatoid arthritis: changes in disease activity, muscle strength and aerobic capacity. *Clin Exp Rheumatol* **6**: 253–260.

National Ankylosing Spondylitis Society (1997) *Research Update*. NASS News.

Thomson A, Skinner A and Piercy J (eds) (1991) Degenerative arthropathies. In: *Tidy's Physiotherapy*, 12th edn. Butterworth Heinemann, Oxford.

9

Orthopaedic Rehabilitation

Aquatic therapy is extremely beneficial for most orthopaedic conditions and can play a vital part in rehabilitation, but what do we mean by orthopaedic conditions? For the purposes of this book, the definition is any common musculo-skeletal dysfunction on which an orthopaedic surgeon is asked to consult. This includes non-surgical conditions such as spinal and other pain, primarily due to musculoskeletal dysfunction or trauma, as well as the traditional areas associated with the orthopaedic surgeon: the treatment of fractures, joint replacement and spinal surgery. This chapter will be divided into three sections: dysfunctions of the spine, the lower limbs and the upper limbs.

Spinal Problems

Back pain, particularly lumbar pain, is extremely common, indeed it accounts for more days off work than any other condition. Almost every-body suffers back pain at some time in their life. This can vary in severity from the vast majority who suffer a few minor twinges which settle within two to three weeks (either spontaneously or with the help of some form of therapy), to the 1–2% whose lives are totally devastated by chronic pain resistant to surgery or therapy. In spite of its frequency, only a very small percent-age of spinal pain sufferers require surgical inter-vention (moreover such intervention is frequently now undertaken by neurosurgeons, not ortho-paedic surgeons). Whilst the statistics on chronic or acute back pain are awesome, the postural and degenerative contribution to it are such that pro-motion of a healthier lifestyle, with positive exer-cise into later life, may in the future be able to prevent much of this misery.

There are, of course, a myriad of factors which can result in back pain, the most important and common of which are postural abnormalities, trauma and degenerative changes. Each of these important categories will be looked at, although in many cases it is not clear which of these three factors actually produces the pain and it may well be a combination of all three. It must not be for-gotten, though, that in a few, fortunately rare cases, back pain can be caused by serious under-lying pathology, such as inflammatory arthritic disease, or cancer. The former has been dealt with in Chapter 8, and the latter falls beyond the remit of this book (although an awareness of it is vital for the physiotherapist, before embarking on treatment of severe back pain of undiagnosed origin).

Postural Abnormalities

A normal spine is a highly complex structure that could be said to be a perfect combination of function and design. Even the best machines can break down, and such a breakdown is more likely if the work a machine is asked to perform differs from that for which it was designed. Chapter 1 discusses the evolution of the body of *Homo sapiens* by a process of natural selection. That selection was based on the lifestyle of early man over hundreds of thousands of years. The demands imposed on a spinal column by that lifestyle would have been very different from those of present-day cultures, which arose in an 'instant' of time, after our anatomical evolution was complete. Sitting would have been minimal, and the main activities would have been walking, squatting, stretching and climbing. Whereas exercise was then essential to collect and hunt for food, nowadays exercise is for many people only a leisure activity. They spend the majority of their waking time sitting down, in the driving seat of a car, in front of a computer or, potentially even more damaging, slouched in front of a television, possibly watching sport instead of participating in it! The very fact that the majority of people suffering with back pain find that the seated posture makes their pain worse, must point to a role of sitting in the cause of the pain in the first place.

But of course not all back pain is due to misplaced inactivity or poor posture. The spine can develop abnormally or unevenly, resulting in deformities such as lordosis and kyphosis, as illustrated in Fig. 9.1.

Fortunately, these abnormalities are usually minor, and rarely cause marked deformity. Spinal deformity used to occur more commonly as a result of paralysis (e.g. polio) or infection (e.g. spinal

Figure 9.1   Abnormalities of the spine.

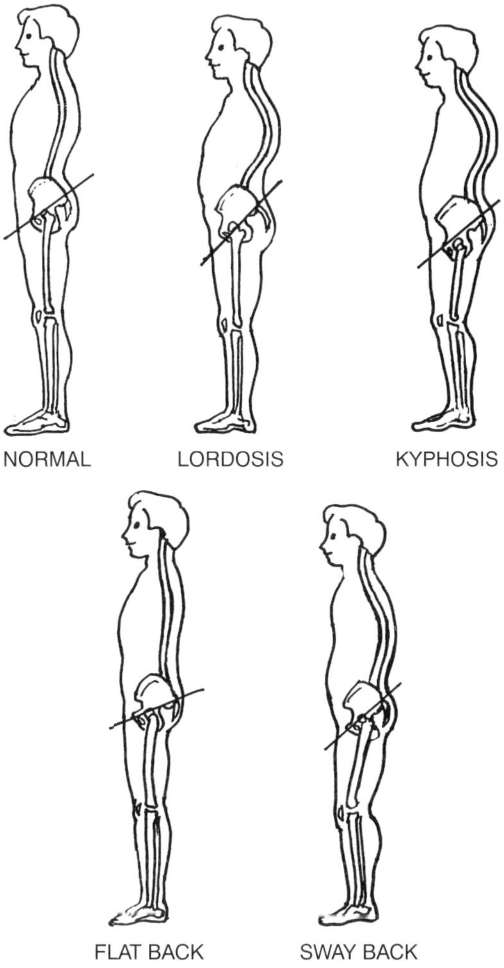

NORMAL   LORDOSIS   KYPHOSIS

FLAT BACK   SWAY BACK

tuberculosis), but such conditions are now almost unknown in Western medicine. These days the development of the above abnormalities is usually spontaneous, and of unknown origin. Severe abnormalities in spines which are still growing will probably require surgical correction, but this is very rare. It is much commoner to find an exaggerated lumbar lordosis which is an extension of a normal posture rather than a pathological condition, or a minor scoliosis perhaps due to compensation for unequal leg length.

IMPLICATIONS FOR AQUATIC THERAPY

For those unfortunate young people who do require surgical intervention, hydrotherapy afterwards is very specialized and will involve a paediatric or orthopaedic hydrotherapist. There is likely to be a lengthy period of immobilization following surgery, and the resultant stiffness and muscle weakness will require mobilization and strengthening when appropriate. The young victims will really appreciate the enhanced freedom of movement which is possible when the constraints of gravity have been removed by immersion.

The majority of adults with a mild degree of spinal curvature are likely to develop secondary degenerative changes. Aquatic therapy for this will be dealt with below, but when dealing with a scoliosis, it may be helpful to stretch out the concave side by unilaterally reaching towards the ceiling. This is one of the few times, in aquatic therapy, when it is necessary to lift an arm out of the water (Fig. 9.2).

It must be remembered that a certain degree of spinal curvature in the anterior/posterior plane is absolutely normal, and kyphosis and lordosis can be looked upon as an exaggeration of the normal spinal curves. (Scoliosis, a sideways curvature, is always an unwanted abnormality.) Those people whose spines are very flat, thereby lacking the normal curves, carry just as much risk of developing backache as those with exaggerated curves. It would be apposite to conjecture that people with perfect posture and deportment are less likely to get back pain without injury, but there is no evidence to support this.

Trauma

While serious spinal trauma, resulting in fractures and possibly paralysis is fortunately rare and beyond the remit of this book, minor trauma to the spine is very common. An obviously traumatic cause is when young persons overextend themselves in the cause of athletic excellence, by getting stretched, or thumped, or forced into a compromising position by other players or a rapid encounter with the ground. The less dramatic, but equally serious scenario is the middle-aged person who bends and twists to get an object from a low place, lifts something heavy or gets out of bed and leans forward over a basin (e.g. to clean their teeth). In all instances there may be a sudden acute pain, or a sensation of 'something giving way', followed by a gradually worsening pain over a period of several hours or overnight.

Speaking as a therapist who has treated thousands of people with low back pain over 35 years, it is not always easy to know precisely which tissues have been damaged, what is the

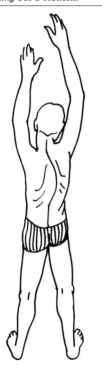

Figure 9.2   Stretching out a scoliosis.

extent of any damage and what will be the likely prognosis. It is extremely rare for such a low back incidence in young people to be a spinal fracture, but the possibility of osteoporotic collapse in older people must always be borne in mind, as must the rare possibility of pathological fractures from underlying metastatic disease (see Glossary). Certainly, the availability of sophisticated scanning devices that allow soft tissue structures to be assessed makes precise diagnosis and prognosis much easier — but only a small percentage of patients who are referred for physiotherapy or hydrotherapy will be subjected to such full investigation.

A person in acute back pain may be unable to stand up properly, either because they cannot straighten the lumbar spine, or because the spine sometimes deviates to one side. The back muscles will probably be in spasm, and this may be unilateral. Muscle spasm may recur not only on the painful side or both sides, but also on the opposite side from the pain and the injury, and may serve as a natural protective, splinting mechanism. Spasm, although possibly useful initially, can become damaging if it continues for more than a day or two. It delivers a compressive force on the spine, the exact opposite of the distraction force applied by traction which usually helps to reduce pain and promote healing. Although the buoyancy effect when standing in water also provides a theoretical 'traction', hydrotherapy during an acute episode is not customarily given in the UK, although it is in North America. Certainly, the treatment of a patient in acute back pain falls into the domain of the medical professional and not the aquatic coach. Too much exercise and/or the wrong exercise can make matters worse.

Most back episodes are probably due to problems with ligaments, facet joints or muscle imbalances, but the trauma may have caused an intervertebral disc to collapse, thereby oozing its central pulpy filling. This may result in subsequent damage to other tissues, of which the most relevant are nerves. The warning that something serious has occurred is the presence of any abnormal neurological signs, i.e. abnormal reflexes, paraesthesia (pins and needles), numbness, and pain referred distal to the injured part (i.e. sciatica, pain in the leg). An acute disc prolapse can also produce muscle weakness in those distal muscles whose nerves have been injured in the spine, and if those muscles are the ones that control the bladder, there can be difficulty in passing water. This last complication is extremely rare, but it requires immediate medical intervention to prevent the real possibility of permanent weakness in the pelvic floor muscles.

To put this into proportion, most back problems, including most disc prolapses, spontaneously resolve. Resolution is helped by 'active rest', i.e. lying down for perhaps 24 hours to 'unload' the damaged part followed by gentle specific exercise to prevent muscle spasm thereafter. This increases the circulation to the area thereby promoting the healing process, as do 'hands-on' techniques such as mobilizing and sometimes re-aligning malaligned segments. Electrotherapy, such as ultrasound or the application of specialized electrical stimulation, can also help to speed up the repair process.

THE ROLE OF AQUATIC THERAPY

An acutely painful back requires rest, as do all other acute inflammations. However, having once suffered such an episode, there is an increased likelihood of a recurrence. Once treatment of the really acute initial episode is over, hydrotherapy may not only speed up resolution, but may help to prevent further such attacks. A disc prolapse is a mechanical problem, and weight and movement through the prolapsed area will frequently make the pain worse. Usually the pain comes on movement – perhaps turning over in bed, or changing from one position to another. The resultant inactivity can cause stiffness and muscle wasting, but any movement that causes pain is undesirable. Water may provide a medium for spinal movements that allows for the initial gentle rehabilitation, but it must always be remembered that too much activity, or exercise in the wrong direction, can further compromise the mechanics and make the patient worse not better. It is therefore imperative to observe the Aquarobics principles, especially those concerning pain and sensible moderation.

In the later stages, aquatic therapy is a wonderful way to regain full flexibility (both muscular and joint), and to strengthen the abdominal muscles which play such an important role in the correct function of the spine. It is also possible to undertake gentle stretching in the water, such as the exercise illustrated in Fig. 9.3, which stretches

Figure 9.3   Hamstring/sciatic stretching.

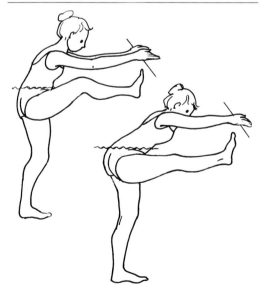

both the sciatic nerve and the hamstring muscles, the tightness of which can predispose to back injury. Indeed, the pool is a perfect place to do this – providing that adequate warnings are given that such stretching can be provocative.

Degenerative Changes

What are the common degenerative changes to the spine? The discs lose bulk with age, the collagen tending to separate and crack and the central nucleus losing fluid and becoming more fibrous. Such changes do not necessarily cause any pain or symptoms. Spondylosis is the syndrome of painful degeneration that occurs between the vertebral bodies and the intervertebral discs. The bodies become 'lipped' and there is a change in mechanics of the discs. This can happen in the lower cervical region where it may result in pain in the arm and/or shoulder, as well as in the lumbar region, where it may result in sciatica.

Other parts of the spinal column are prone to degenerative changes. Ligaments may become contracted and weakened and the facet joints may succumb to the classic OA changes of thickened capsule, and osteophyte formation. This will reduce the space in the intervertebral foramina causing pressure on nerve roots and severe pain either locally or distally in the distribution of the nerve root. Severe degenerative changes in the lumbar area can lead to a condition known as spinal stenosis, when the foramina of the canals carrying nerve roots become severely restricted. The condition, previously untreatable, can now be alleviated by microsurgery. The final tissues that can be affected, are the meningeal sleeve around the spinal cord and nerve roots. The increased pressure caused by the above degenerative changes can result in chronic, but none-theless very painful, inflammation.

Although disc prolapses have been categorized above as traumatic in origin, there are a considerable number which happen as a result of generalized degenerative changes to the spine. Perhaps the final prolapse is like 'the straw that broke the camel's back', in that degenerative changes caused a mechanical weakness, and some other relatively minor force was sufficient to cause the final 'unbalancing'. Indeed, the continued minor trauma could have been due to poor posture or bad working habits, thereby meaning that a disc prolapse may be due to one or more of the following combinations: poor posture, trauma or degenerative changes. This perhaps is a rationale for the holistic approach to treatment. It is necessary to treat the injured region, to re-align posture and to enhance the movement ability of the whole body. It also explains the maxim 'use it or lose it', as under-use inactivity throughout the range of movement is one of the many factors involved in degenerative changes.

Aquatic Exercise for Back Pain

I. ACUTE STAGE

As indicated above, therapy when immersed, for those in acute, severe back pain, should only be given in a medical context. The main objective of such hydrotherapy is to reduce and/or centralize pain. If such objectives are achieved, then more proactive therapy, such as muscular stabilization or gentle restoration of pain-free movement can then be carefully initiated.

When immersed in a vertical position, buoyancy

produces a slight traction force on the spine. If the pool is deep enough, this can be enhanced by using buoyancy aids under the arms, possibly whilst weighing down the feet. There is a real risk of an increase in pain on coming out of the water, as gravity re-asserts normal weight through the spine. Also, dressing and undressing are difficult for patients with really severe problems. Because of these factors, plus the fact that most hydrotherapy pools are not deep enough, immersion traction is not often practised in the UK. In my practice, acute back pain patients have been immersed only a handful of times – and then only because dry therapy did not seem to be effective, the patients requested it, and there was an urgency in the timescale necessitating slight risk-taking.

In North America. it is more common to immerse acute patients. This is done either vertically, supported supine on floats or, with the help of a mask and snorkel, in the prone position.

2. SUBACUTE STAGE

The subacute stage is the intervening period between an acute episode (which does not normally last more than 3 weeks) and the chronic recovery period thereafter. Aquatic exercise is appropriate for some people in the subacute stage, but probably still under overall medical supervision. However, whilst it is appropriate for those people whose pain diminishes on activity, it could cause an increase in pain if the wrong exercise or excessive exercise is given. In order to establish who can start early aquatic rehabilitation and what precisely that exercise should include, it is necessary to take a detailed history of the pain and the precipitating and alleviating factors, and to carry out a careful physical examination. Such careful case taking and examination is beyond the remit of the aquatic coach, but in certain establishments, such coaches may conduct sessions under the direction of therapists or other medical or allied professionals.

The likely aims and objectives of treatment at this stage will be to reduce pain (actively by exercise or passively by positioning), and to start rehabilitation by strengthening appropriate muscles (trunk and abdominal) and increasing the range of affected joints. Table 9.1 suggests a few exercises that would help achieve these objectives. Many others can be found in Section IV.

3. CHRONIC STAGE AND PROPHYLACTIC EXERCISES

By far the majority of people who require aquatic therapy or exercise for a recovering or a chronic back problem will fall into this category. Such exercises are also appropriate for those who have actually recovered, and are therefore free from pain, as it is hoped that continuing indefinitely will reduce the possibility of further episodes.

As such people will now be able to work faster and harder, such exercises can be performed in the cooler temperatures of a swimming pool.

The objectives of aquatic exercise for people in this group are to maintain or increase flexibility, to maintain or increase strength of all trunk and limb muscles, to enhance fitness and well-being by aerobic training, and to provide enjoyment. Most of the exercises in Section IV, Parts A and B, will help achieve these aims. Generally speaking the ones selected in Table 9.1 are easier than the ones in Table 9.2. The former could therefore be used in the warm-up section for those with chronic problems, and the harder exercises (and others from Section IV) can be incorporated into the strengthening and mobility sections of the work-out.

If people are to continue attending (which is a prerequisite for the prophylactic objective) it is important that aquatic exercise is enjoyable and not boring. In order to achieve this, it is helpful to have lively music, and a programme which varies from week to week. Once it becomes the same old set routine, it is in danger of not only becoming boring, but of not being sufficiently challenging in order to maintain the 'training' goals implicit in the objectives.

Lower Limb Dysfunction

Arguably, the region of the body that has the most to gain from aquatic rehabilitation, is the lower quadrant. The more common orthopaedic conditions that afflict the pelvis and leg will be examined in the light of any implication regarding aquatic exercise, starting from the pelvis and working footwards.

It will be assumed that fractures or soft tissue damage are the result of trauma. It should be mentioned, though, that some fractures are caused by a cancer, either a primary or secondary. This, fortunately, is extremely rare, but will have implications for aquatic therapy. A patient with a cancer-related problem will be having other therapy, and this (or the disease) may make them too ill to go into a pool, at least in the early stages. Moreover, radiotherapy is sometimes incompatible with immersion of any kind (even washing the affected part), for a certain length of time. Obviously it is imperative to work in close cooperation with oncologists, radiologists and the entire medical team. Cancer will not be dealt with any further

Table 9.1
Exercises in the subacute stage of back pain

Objective	Exercise	Notes	Exercise no.
Reduction of pain	Forwards (heel–toe) walking	Chest-deep	90
	Diagonal arm reaches	Chest-deep	2
	Corkscrew	Chest-deep	3
	Twists	May need support	35
	Cycling	May need support	25
	Helicopters	With floats	34
Increase strength (a) postural stability	Leg swinging		70
			83
	Small range paddle corkscrew	Shoulder-high water	37
	Backwards (toe–heel) walking	Chest-deep	91
(b) abdominals	Parts and crossovers	More advanced	39
	Toe-out curls		26
	Alternate toe-out curls		27
Increase range of movement	Bumps and grinds		12
	Belly dance		11
	Spoon corkscrew		36
	Side bends		21
	Half figurehead	With care	16
	Pancake tucks		30
	Hamstring stretch		102
	Wall squats		17
	Pike squats and stretch		109
	Wall kneels		18

in this book, apart from hydrotherapy to the shoulder following a mastectomy (see below).

There are a number of other general points to make about injury. (i) Any trauma that is suffi- cient to fracture a normal, healthy bone will involve a certain amount of soft tissue injury. (ii) The healing rates of different tissues vary, and are in direct proportion to the amount of the

Table 9.2
Exercises for the chronic stage of back pain and prophylaxis

Objective	Exercise	Notes	Exercise no.
Increase range of movement	Diagonal arm reaches		2
	Side bends with reaches		21
	V-shapes		40
	Rowing		15
	The figurehead		16
	Wall kneels		18
	Facet pushes		24
Increase in trunk strength	Loaded leg swinging	Load with ankle floats	70, 83
	Sea-horsing	Requires trunk stability	51
	Paddle corkscrew	Hold float to load	37
	Golf swings	Hold a flipper	50
	Deep water running		99
	Pancake tucks and/or flippers	Can load with flippers	30
Increased aerobic capacity	Running on the spot		
	Spotty dog		
	Spotty dog with head still		
	Part jumps and crossovers		
	Elbow to knee runs		
	Tuck jumps		
	Frog jumps		
	Clap under thigh jumps		
Enhanced enjoyment	Floating relaxation		112–114

blood supplied to that tissue. (iii) Bones have a good blood supply: when a bone is fractured there is substantial blood loss; generally speaking, the larger the bone, the greater the haemorrhage. In fact, 25% of people who fracture their femurs die because of the physiological shock caused by the loss of blood. (iv) Ligaments have a comparatively poor blood supply, and therefore sprains (i.e. torn ligaments) take longer to heal properly than fractures of bones. (v) Performing normal functional movements without limping and without pain is a powerful form of therapy. It is often possible to achieve a relatively normal gait in water long before this can be done on dry land, without walking aids like crutches. Not only are there physical advantages to this, such as the limitation of muscle wasting, the prevention of joint stiffness, and an increase in local circulation that has the effect of promoting healing, but the psychological boost of being able to do 'normal' things like walk, without requiring mechanical aids or feeling pain, is a great facilitator of the therapy process.

The Aquarobics approach to hydrotherapy is holistic, involving functional movement patterns and multiple joint activity. It is therefore probable that patients undergoing aquatic rehabilitation for dysfunctions of the pelvis, hips, femurs, knees or ankles, will be on fairly similar programmes. Specific exercises for each condition will not therefore be given, but indications for particular exercises will be given in Table 9.3, classified according to the effort the patient can expend, i.e. early, gentle rehabilitation; moderate effort in the middle stages and 'tough' rehabilitation in the final stage.

The Pelvis

Fractures of the pelvic bones are fortunately uncommon, but are included here because hydrotherapy is so helpful in the subsequent rehabilitation. They happen as the result of trauma to the lower trunk from falling or crushing, most commonly from road traffic accidents, but also quite characteristically from falling down mountains (on the ski slopes or when mountaineering). If the fracture line falls within the hip or sacro-iliac joint, then the eventual result may be somewhat less favourable.

The most vulnerable part of the pelvis is at the front — the pubic rami — but if the force is sufficient, a fracture can happen at any part. Indeed, multiple fractures of the pelvis are not uncommon. Fractures are classified as stable or unstable, and their management will depend on the number, site and stability of the lesions. It must be remembered that any force great enough to fracture the pelvic bones will probably have also injured the contents of the pelvis and abdomen; such patients might initially have been very ill. Also, it is not uncommon to have additional associated fractures in the femur, the spine or elsewhere in the body.

After the period of bed rest is over, the patient will probably be sent home on crutches, thereby reducing the weight that goes through the fracture site when walking. Hydrotherapy for a fractured pelvis may be started early, before the fracture has united. Because a lot of force is necessary to fracture a pelvis, the other injuries incurred may delay the onset of hydrotherapy. At the other end of the spectrum, it is possible to have a minor, undisplaced fracture (usually of the pelvic radii) which is fairly simple to rehabilitate. Providing that the patient's general condition is satisfactory, then hydrotherapy is very helpful and should dramatically hasten the rehabilitation period. The benefit is both physical and psychological and provides an early opportunity for pain-free locomotion. Patients may be suffering from post-traumatic stress, and it is therefore all the more important to make the immersion experience positive and enjoyable, to alert them to the possibility that they will be able to walk normally again. The ability to remove the fear of disability following an injury is a very powerful positive aspect of aquatic rehabilitation.

IMPLICATIONS FOR AQUATIC THERAPY

When dealing with a disunited fracture, aquatic therapy should initially be in water that is chest- or shoulder-deep to minimize weight bearing. However, if walking in such water is without pain, then it may be possible to move into shallower water, so that a small amount of weight goes through the damaged part, which may help to promote healing.

The objectives of hydrotherapy following a fractured pelvis are to facilitate healing and aid the return of normal functional movement patterns, particularly all forms of walking. This involves targeting other tissues too: mobilizing joints of the spine and limbs within pain-free limits, strengthening musculature in the region to improve balance and coordination, and providing an opportunity for relaxation and enjoyment.

Hip Replacement Arthroplasty

Total hip replacement (THR) might be considered one of the main success stories of Western medicine. The operation involves replacing one or both of the articulating surfaces at the hip joint, namely the head and neck of the femur and the 'cup' of the acetabulum in the pelvis. There are many different types of arthroplasties. The original successful one was developed in the 1970s by Charnley, but a host of alternatives have since been developed. The procedure is used to replace a worn joint, in rheumatoid or osteoarthritis, and sometimes after a fracture of the neck of the femur (see below). Although widely practised, and generally very successful in relieving pain and improving function, this operation is not without risk. As well as the usual risks of any major surgery, namely cardiovascular complications or infection, there are the specific risks of disloca-

tion (fortunately very rare) and the more likely risk of the components failing. The average life of a hip arthroplasty is 10 years; a few fail soon after surgery whereas others will give no problems for over 20 years. Because of the technical difficulties of revising a failed arthroplasty, surgeons are reluctant to perform these on younger patients who are not only likely to ask more from their new joint, but who are more likely to outlive the normal life of the artificial joint. Usually the components are cemented into place, to allow for speedy weight bearing. In younger patients, however, the arthroplasty may be installed without cement, to allow for easier revision when the time eventually comes. In such instances, the patients are not allowed to take any weight through their new hips for a period of about six weeks, and must therefore rely on crutches for up to three months.

HYDROTHERAPY FOLLOWING A HIP REPLACEMENT

It is very difficult to generalize on the specifics of post-operative treatment, because each surgeon has his/her own post-operative protocol. Indeed, there are a few surgeons who ban post-operative physiotherapy and/or hydrotherapy, presumably in the belief that over-active therapy is more likely to cause joint dislocation. Certainly over-active therapy too soon is potentially dangerous. In order to insert the prosthesis, the surgeon will have had to dislocate the old joint by putting the hip into a position of extreme flexion and adduction, thereby stretching the capsule. Therefore, immediately after the operation, the leg is placed into abduction and extension and, once mobility can start, the flexed adducted position should be avoided, and any crossing of the legs.

The aims of hydrotherapy will initially be to improve the walking pattern, and to strengthen muscles in the region which were not only weakened by years of disease, but which have been cut by the surgeon's knife. Real aquatic resistance training to strength will probably not start until about 4–6 weeks after the operation, depending on the surgeon's protocol. However, one of the best results I have ever seen following arthroplasty is my husband's case. Because we have a hydrotherapy pool at home, he was able to exercise daily once discharged from hospital. The surgeon did an excellent job, but the regular hydrotherapy really contributed to the successful outcome.

Any exercise that involves crossing the leg, or forcing hip flexion has the potential of causing a dislocation, and must therefore be avoided. It is better to teach walking in slight abduction initially.

As it is impossible to keep pool water totally sterile, it is important to protect the wound as much as possible. There are water-tight sterile dressings available.

Initially, it is common practice to ban sitting on low chairs and this includes toilet seats, so as to limit hip flexion. It is therefore necessary to ensure that the chairs and toilet in the changing rooms are high enough, or that there is a 'raise', available to fit where required. It is common for patients to wear compression stockings, and these may be full-length. Patients will be unable to cope with these by themselves, without leaning forward and over-stretching the hip. Help must therefore be available for dressing and undressing.

Fractures of the Femur

Fractures of the femur can be broadly categorized into those in the upper end (most commonly by far, through the neck of the femur), those of the femoral shaft, and those which occasionally occur at the lower end and may involve the knee joint.

Generally, fractures of the femoral neck happen as a result of osteoporosis, and so usually occur in the elderly. As already indicated, they are potentially life-threatening, mainly because of haemorrhage. Depending on the precise circumstances of the fracture, treatment is either by internal fixation (when a long nail is inserted through the medullary space of the bone), or by partial (or total) hip replacement. In either instance, early mobilization is desirable, and the patients will be mobilized as soon as their general condition permits. In some units, where hydrotherapy is available, the wound will be dressed so as to render it waterproof, and hydrotherapy will be commenced just a few days after surgery.

This is in contrast to subtrochanteric fractures, and fractures of the femoral shaft, which usually happen to younger adults, in velocity or impact accidents such as those involving motorbikes. They take much longer to rehabilitate, as they require a period of bed rest for up to three months, with the leg placed in mechanical traction. After that time, hydrotherapy is one useful treatment modality, but intensive regular physiotherapy will also be necessary if full pre-injury performance is to be reached.

Total Knee Replacement Arthroplasty

Total knee replacement (TKR) is not yet as successful as that at the hip joint. This is probably because the mechanics around the knee, being a hinge joint, are very complicated and the components are likely to fail. Moreover, the joint is more superficial, and this might explain the incidence of infection. Usually, the patella is left in place, and the patello-femoral joint can cause pain at a later stage. Finally, it is sometimes difficult to regain the expected range of movement. It is hoped that full extension will be achieved, but flexion is often only around 90°. Although this amount of flexion is sufficient for most functional activities, a bit more is desirable.

Nonetheless, this operation can dramatically improve the lifestyle of a person who had been prevented, by pain, from going out and leading a normal life. Sometimes, more or less overnight, the pain and the accompanying depression can simply disappear. Being able to walk more or less normally in water is not only a great psychological boost, but helps restore function, range and strength. Sometimes hydrotherapy is started just a few days after surgery, but this may have to wait until the patient is home. At this time they are probably walking with the help of only one or two canes, but protocols vary enormously from surgeon to surgeon and from country to country.

FACTORS TO CONSIDER IN HYDROTHERAPY

The same factors relating to sterility and help with dressing and undressing will apply, as to those who have had a THR (see above). Moreover, the aims of therapy will be virtually the same: to restore function, particularly walking, to strengthen the muscles in the region and increase the range of movement in the new joint, as determined by the surgeon.

Fractures Around the Knee

Fractures around the knee can happen at any age, and the eventual outcome depends on many fac-

tors, including the precise location, the severity of the fracture and the age of the patient. The fracture may be at the lower end of the femur, and this will probably also involve damage to one of the collateral ligaments of the knee, the upper end of the tibia or fibula or to the patella. Treatment is by reduction (i.e. 'straightening out' the fracture), followed by immobilization in a full-leg cast or, alternatively, by internal fixation. The latter method has the great advantage that the knee and ankle joints do not become so stiff.

Hydrotherapy, when the time is right, is particularly helpful in either case, as walking in water is an excellent way of regaining movement in the knee joint, as well as improving the ability to walk on dry land. Indeed, if all those people who had been immobilized in a cast were instructed, from the day after their cast was removed, to walk in a swimming pool, in chest-high water, there is a strong likelihood that incidence of subsequent complications, such as Sudeck's atrophy or degenerative changes, would be dramatically reduced. Aquatic exercise does of course consist of much more than just walking in water. Ideas for specific exercises will be found in Table 9.3.

Other Injuries to the Knee

The knee joint is surely the most frequently injured joint in the body. There are probably two reasons for this: (i) it is a very complex, inherently unstable joint that relies only on ligaments and muscles for its internal fixation, and (ii) it is particularly prone to injury in activities which involve a sideways force being exerted on a flexed knee – a situation frequently found when skiing, and playing most contact sports. These injuries can take a long time to heal.

A frequent sequela of such ligamentous trauma to the knee is the requirement for microsurgery. This is now a very sophisticated and precise

Table 9.3
Suggested exercises for lower limb dysfunction

Objective	Exercise	Notes	Exercise no.
To reduce swelling	Any vertical exercise	Hydrostatic pressure and muscle pump	
To improve gait	The changes	A useful warm-up	1
	Weight transfer with reaches	Variations on lunging	66
	Forward (heel–toe) walking	Reciprocal arm and leg gait	90
	Backwards (toe–heel) walking	The opposite arm goes back with the leg	91
	Walking sideways	With or without flexed knees	92
	Diagonal reaches		2
	Braiding		94
To strengthen muscles	Leg swinging	Make harder with a foot float	70, 83
	Shallow squats	Requires shallow water	85
	Cossackski's	Care! Not to be done if knee unstable	89
	Quads and hamstring pumps		79, 81
	Wall knee rises	Requires a rail and not too sensitive knee	77
	Running		95, 96, 99
	Step-ups		77
	Fast flipper walking		98
To increase range in joints	Step lunges		67
	Wall pushes		68
	Rises		82
	Cycling		25
	Steam engine circles		65
	Superglue exercise	Must keep the trunk raised	73
	Vertical and horizontal scissors		28 74
	Wall squats and kneels		17, 18
	Calf, quads and hamstring stretches		101, 102, 103

method of investigating and repairing internal damage to the menisci, or the cruciate ligaments. Hydrotherapy is very useful one or two days after such surgery, to reduce swelling and restore normal movement.

Another problem around the knee is pain associated with knee bending, felt at the front of the knee joint, under the patella. Chondromalacia patella is the name for the syndrome which results in a softening of the posterior surface of the patella. It is usually associated with an imbalance of the quadriceps muscles, the vastus medialis being weak, so that the patella impinges on the surface of the femur instead of tracking centrally straight up its groove. Treatment may be conservative, using strapping and muscle re-education techniques to re-programme the quadriceps, or by arthroscopic surgery which shaves the damaged surface of the patella. Hydrotherapy may be useful in either instance.

Fractures and Sprains of the Ankle and Foot

Injuries to the ankle and foot are fairly common, and aquatic rehabilitation should theoretically reduce the risk of re-injury or other complication. A torsional force applied to the ankle can sprain either or both of the collateral ligaments, or fracture either or both of the tibial or fibular malleoli. Any one or more of these events can compromise the integrity of the mortice that should provide stability to the ankle and foot. If the injury requires immobilization, then additional stiffness will develop.

The muscles acting in the region are very complicated, and activities such as balancing on one foot require a high degree of coordination. This is achieved through 'proprioception', which is the awareness of position, movement and balance of

the body as a whole or any of its parts, which comes from the fine neurological control of movement by reflex afferent and efferent pathways. Like other motor skills, balance has to be practised, or the ability to perform is diminished. Thus, an injury to the ankle or foot can severely affect the subsequent ability of the body to control balance and coordination. In order to 'train' balance ability, it is necessary to get to the point of losing balance, then re-gaining it. Out of the water, this is potentially hazardous, as an inability to balance may well result in another fall and further injury.

Aquatic exercise is an excellent way of improving this ability as the water slows down movements, giving time to transfer weight and re-adjust the centre of gravity. It is also possible to practise different walking techniques, such as on tip-toe, on the heels, on the insides or the outsides of the feet. Such unorthodox postures would be painful, and possibly impossible to do when not immersed, because of the pain caused by weight going through sensitive injured tissues.

OBJECTIVES OF AQUATIC EXERCISE FOR DYSFUNCTION OF THE LOWER QUADRANT

Support and locomotion are probably the most important functions of the lower quadrant, so aquatic exercises should aim to improve walking ability, which is an amalgamation of these functions. This may be done initially, by simply standing in chest-high water, with a wide base, and going through the motions of transferring weight from one foot to the other. When this is easy, locomotion exercises can be commenced, with the aim of facilitating as normal a gait pattern as possible. Reducing any swelling is also an objective.

Other more specific objectives are to strengthen

all the muscles of the lower leg, but especially those near the site of dysfunction. It is equally important to restore the normal range of movement to all joints in the limb, but both these objectives may take some sessions to achieve. The experience should also be enjoyable, because this helps enormously to dispel anxiety. If rehabilitation is fun, compliance with instructions and positive outcomes are much more likely. The exercises listed below are primarily for the legs. There is no reason, though, why appropriate arm movements should not also be happening at the same time (apart, of course, from those horizontal exercises which involve holding on).

Upper Quadrant Dysfunction

Anatomical Considerations

The shoulder is not just one joint, but a highly complex series of joints involving the humerus, the clavicle, the scapula and the chest wall. If one had to opt for a single point of contact between the upper limb and the trunk, it would be the sternoclavicular joint, which can be felt to move as the arm elevates. However, that joint rarely demonstrates dysfunctions, whereas the glenohumeral joint frequently does. It is a ball and socket joint, and the most mobile joint in the body and hence prone to being dislocated. The scapula articulates with the clavicle, making an arch above the ball of the humerus through which pass tendons which are prone to being squashed. Indeed, the area around the shoulder could be looked upon as a complex junction of tendons, blood vessels and nerves, rather like a complicated railway junction.

In order for the arm to be fully raised above the head, the scapula must glide around the chest wall. This all requires the most elaborate muscular coordination with precision timing; it is not at all surprising that it sometimes goes wrong. Finally, all of the above-mentioned structures are close to the cervical spine and its departing nerve roots and nerves. Shoulder dysfunctions frequently have a cervical component, and vice versa.

In addition to the mechanical impingement, muscle imbalance and coordination problems mentioned above, fractures are fairly common in the area. Whereas fractures of the clavicle are relatively unimportant and usually regain normal function fairly easily, fractures of the humerus are harder to rehabilitate. The area is prone to degenerative changes and soft-tissue impingement of tendons, which then result in extreme pain and an inability to raise the arm. A 'frozen shoulder' is a stiff and painful shoulder, but it is not really a diagnosis; it is rather a definition of a symptom. The underlying reason for the stiffness could be due to a number of causes: tendon impingement, fractures, inflammation of the joint capsule or the subacromial bursa, or other, rarer causes.

Shoulder problems can be extremely painful. Sometimes, in the acute stage, the pain is even experienced at rest. Immersion exercise is not appropriate at this time – the acute inflammation needs to settle, and only rest, analgesic anti-inflammatory electrotherapy or gentle handling techniques can be used. Once the condition has settled, then gentle immersion can be tried. It should be remembered, though, that there will be no real effect from hydrostatic pressure, because the shoulder joints are too near the surface to engender any significant force.

Immersion is particularly appropriate for resolving problems around the shoulder, as buoyancy permits movements that would be too painful out of the water, because of the complicated

Table 9.4
Suggested exercises for upper limb dysfunction
It is important that none of these exercises should cause an increase in pain

Objective	Exercise	Notes	Exercise no.
To reduce pain	The changes	All shoulder movement to be slow and gentle	1
	Shoulder shrugs	Find what reduces the pain by trial and error	41
	Walking	Keep the arms down, and only minimal movement	90 91 93
To improve function	The changes	A useful warm-up	1
	Elbow circling	Neck-high water	47
	Biceps/triceps curl	Without weights	55
	Forward (heel–toe) walking	Reciprocal arm–leg gait	90
	Backwards (toe–heel) walking	Toe–heel and opposite arm	91
	Walking sideways	With arm floating up and flexed knees	92 93
	Diagonal reaches	Slightly less diagonal and more forwards	2
	Shallow squats	Let the arms float up as the legs go down, firstly into flexion, then into abduction	85
	Running	With reciprocal arm movement	95, 96
	Sea-horsing	Using the arms to help with propulsion	51
	Cutting a diamond	Get the back of the hands on the buttock	45
To improve aerobic fitness	Any aerobic exercise	Must be within comfortable range of movement	

Table 9.4 (continued)

Suggested exercises for upper limb dysfunction

It is important that none of these exercises should cause an increase in pain

Objective	Exercise	Notes	Exercise no.
To strengthen muscles	Biceps pump	Made harder with a small buoyant float, e.g. an ankle float or arm band with only a little air	59
	Diagonal reaches	Possibly with equipment	2
	Triceps pump	Take care that the starting position is not provocative. Progress as for biceps pump	60
	Pectoral and low trap squeezes	If painless, can use minimum buoyancy weight; non-buoyant weights might overwork the abductors	62
	Hand figure-of-eight	Keep the elbows wedged; this works the shoulder rotators. Can progress to paddles or small flippers	48
	Tennis swings	A plastic bat (with holes in it) will increase load	49
	Golf swings	Two-handed, using the arms as a club	50
	Wall press-ups	Triceps and biceps press-ups	52
To increase range in joints	Corkscrew	Extending the back arm	3
	Stride jumps	Only when nearly better. Cross arms in front and behind with the elbows straight	

Table 9.4 (continued)
Suggested exercises for upper limb dysfunction
It is important that none of these exercises should cause an increase in pain

Objective	Exercise	Notes	Exercise no.
	Figure-of-eight	A whole-body movement with weight transference	87
	Side circles	Similar; may involve coming out of the water	58
	Arm walking	Better not to impose a rhythm	46
	Swim kicks		71
	Side bends with reaches	With full weight transfer and lunging	21

interplay of muscles, some of which might be dysfunctional. To benefit from the buoyancy, the shoulder joints must be immersed. If the water is too shallow to permit this, then the knees must be flexed to adopt a semi-squatting posture, or a plastic stool, or armless chair can be placed in the pool and the exercises conducted in the seated position.

Factors to Consider with Aquatic Therapy

It is suggested that upper body and arm exercise starts by warming up the muscles of the shoulder girdle, and this is best achieved by doing several of the shoulder shrugging exercises, preferably with the hands down at the sides. When standing (preferably with a wide base for additional stability) the arm will more or less float into the horizontal position. As it is buoyancy rather than active muscle work which is bringing up the arm, there is a much reduced chance of impinging the rotator cuff tendons and hence producing pain. As this movement is frequently painful when done non-immersed, it is a comforting one with which to start glenohumeral movement. The active part of the exercise can then be the pushing downwards, so as to get the hands to touch the thighs.

Implications for Aquatic Therapy

Symmetrical exercises, or those that involve using the arms in reciprocal movement to the legs, are recommended not only because they are more functional, but because, by working on the whole body, they divert the concentration from the painful part, and so reduce the fear.

If trying to elevate the arm above 90°, whilst keeping it immersed, or on the surface of the water, it is necessary to be in a semi-recumbent supine or side-lying position. An example of an

Figure 9.4 'Swimming' exercise.

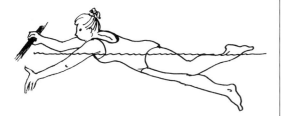

activity which combines both these points would be lying more or less prone, holding on to the side with one hand, while the other hand is pushing the body away from the wall, and helping to maintain it in the horizontal position (see Fig. 9.4). It is relatively unimportant which hand does what, and the choice may depend on pain and range of movement but, ideally, the hands should 'swop over' halfway through the exercise. The exercise could then be either a simple crawl-legs kicking, or prone tucks. The latter is much more demanding on the arms.

The primary objective should be to minimize pain. Once that is achieved then functional movements can be started, with the aim of increasing the range of movement and building up strength in the region. If at all possible, some of the exercises should be performed at sufficient intensity so as to improve the aerobic functioning. This will not only engender a feeling of well-being, but may release some endorphins which will reduce the pain. Table 9.4 gives some relevant exercises. However, because all exercises should be 'holistic', if possible and not confined to any one dysfunctional region, then the number of potentially helpful exercises is enormous. Providing the body is moved in natural patterns, and that no pain is produced, then the outcome of a session is likely to be not only beneficial to the functioning of the injured part, but to have engendered an overall feeling of well-being.

10

Aquarobics for the Overweight

There are two kinds of overweight people; the few who are happy with their shape, and the vast majority who would dearly love to inhabit a thinner body. But, even for those trying to lose just a few pounds, the process is not easy. Can Aquarobics assist in weight loss? Although a serious study has not been undertaken, there are many anecdotal reports that regular aquatic exercise can reduce weight in the overweight – providing, of course, that there is not a corresponding increase in calorific intake. There are sound theoretical reasons why this should be so, but it is necessary to have a brief review of physiology to explain them.

Relevant Physiology

Firstly, it is perhaps stating the obvious to say that the surplus tissue in overweight people is the fat which is laid down as adipose tissue. This is found subcutaneously all over the body, particularly in the abdomen. It must not be thought of as 'dollops of lard' because, like all other body tissues, it is supplied with blood vessels and nerve endings, essential for its function as a reservoir of fuel. This is not the only function of fat in the body; it is an insulator, a cushion for internal organs, and a moulder of body shape, particularly

in females. However, excess fat is not only aesthetically undesirable (at least in contemporary Western society), it is a health hazard.

To some extent, whether or not a person is technically defined as 'obese' will depend on their height, body fat content and age. A current method of definition is by using the Body Mass Index (BMI; Valadian, 1992). A simple index of weight-for-height has been devised. It is calculated as follows:

$$BMI = \frac{Weight\ (kg)}{Height^2\ (m^2)}$$

The BMI of an adult of 70 kg with a height of 175 cm is

$$\frac{70}{(1.75 \times 1.75)} = 22.9$$

The international accepted ranges of BMIs are as follows:

Underweight	< 18.5
Normal	18.9–24.9
Overweight	25.0–29.9
Obesity	30.0–39.9
Extremely obese	≥ 40

Excess fat deposition is the inevitable result of excess calorific intake. The energy-expenditure side of the calorie equation is essentially made up of two components — basal metabolism and muscle activity. Much of the former reflects the more-or-less constant energy demands of organs such as liver, brain and kidneys, with muscle, at rest, probably only accounting for less than 30% of the metabolic rate. Whilst it is possible that increased muscle tone and certain biochemical adaptations to training might increase this contribution in the fit person, it is only by increasing muscle work that you can really 'burn off' those excess calories. And it is quite depressing to calculate how long and how hard you need to work daily in order to have a significant effect on your overall calorie expenditure!

In starvation, or *very* prolonged exercise, all your body's energy stores — liver and muscle glycogen, fat and muscle protein are eventually mobilized and burned. In the case of short-term exercise, however, the kind of work you do influences fuel selection.

In Chapter 2 (Exercise Physiology) it was mentioned that there are several different kinds of muscle fibres. All muscles are made up of two or more different fibre types, arranged in 'packages', each with its own specific kind of innervation. However, in any particular muscle there is a preponderance of either fast-twitch or slow-twitch fibres, depending partly on the kind of work that the muscle normally performs, genetic predisposition and training. Fast-twitch muscle fibres have anaerobic metabolism, fuelled by glucose units from muscle glycogen (or blood sugar, replenished by liver glycogen), readily available for an instant response, but quickly depleted and therefore unable to be maintained for very long. Slow-twitch muscles, on the other hand, can be either sugar or fat burning. After exercising for some time, if the exercise is maintained at a high level, the immediate blood, muscle and liver glycogen

stores will be depleted, and the dominant fuel will become fat. It is therefore reckoned to be aerobic metabolism which burns fat and which, eventually, will lead to weight reduction.

Those muscles in the body which have to work all the time to maintain the upright position against gravity, namely the extensor muscle groups, tend to have a preponderance of slow-twitch, aerobic fibres. The way to 'burn' fat, is therefore to indulge in a moderately high level of whole body activity for 20–30 minutes or longer. In other words, to switch to aerobic metabolism after the glycogen has been depleted, and to do this by using the main muscle groups of the body, especially the extensors. Such activity is difficult to achieve on dry land for somebody who is already seriously overweight. There are three main reasons for this: (i) the obvious mechanical strain to joints and muscles because of the additional weight-bearing forces through delicate articular cartilage, ligaments, tendons and muscles, which predispose to injury. Moreover, obese people are frequently unaccustomed to exercising and have not developed the skills necessary to prevent injury. (ii) Subcutaneous fat acts as an insulator, and there is therefore a possibility of hyperthermia on working aerobically for any length of time. (iii) For the above reasons, it is quite unusual for seriously overweight people to be seen working aerobically. There is therefore the further implication that they are 'unfit', and this means that they are cardiovascularly at risk. Adipose tissues, which may account for upwards of 40% of the total 'person', has a rich blood supply, thereby putting even more load through the cardiovascular system. Arteries are prone to fatty deposits which can lead to cardiac infarcts and strokes. Hyperthermia will impose an additional strain on the cardiovascular system.

Why Exercise in Water?

Aquatic exercise is much safer for those who are overweight because the risk of physical injury to the musculoskeletal system is dramatically reduced. Indeed, one could say that such people have an advantage over slimmer people because of the additional buoyancy causing less weight to go through the knees and feet. Moreover, because heat is dispersed in the water at a much greater rate than when non-immersed – the risk of hyperthermia is much reduced, provided that the water is cool enough. These factors combine to give aquatic exercise a reduced risk of cardiovascular insult. It is also likely to be more effective than dry exercise, simply because a higher work intensity is easier to achieve in the water.

How to Lose Weight

The only way to lose weight is to eat less calories than are required for everyday activities and normal metabolism, so as to start to burn off some of the surplus fat. This will happen a little more quickly if also undertaking a regime consisting of moderate aerobic activity. However, drastic calorific reduction combined with strenuous exercise could damage muscle fibres, which require a certain amount of protein to increase their number and size.

The Aquarobic way to lose weight is to use **sensible moderation**. Reduce calorific input. Virtually cut out fat, but remember that many convenience 'healthy foods' have a high hidden fat content, so read the labels. Eat plenty of fresh fruit and vegetables. Cut out sugar, and virtually cut out alcohol. Remember to drink a lot, but water is the best! Protein is actually very calorific, so only have enough to fulfil the body's needs, but remember that there must be sufficient (around

40 g/day) to cope with the normal replacement of cells, which will be increased a little by the increase in overall metabolism caused by exercise.

It is better to lose weight slowly and steadily, as 'crash' diets tend to have a rebound effect afterwards. In fact, the sensible moderation rule works just as well for dieting as it does for Aquarobics.

Aquatic Exercise to Help Weight Loss

Factors to Consider When Exercising Aquatically

There are a few special considerations when planning aquatic exercise or hydrotherapy for the overweight. Firstly, when dealing with those who are seriously overweight, it is important to remember that their cardiovascular system may already be under strain. All exercise must start off slowly and gently, and gradually intensify, observing the Aquarobics principle of sensible moderation.

Ideally, the water should be chest-high to minimize risk of injury, and should be between 26 and 29 °C. This temperature encourages activity to keep warm. If the pool temperature is much above this, as for example in a hydrotherapy pool, and the exercise intensity is moderate, then there is a potential risk of hyperthermia. Clients must therefore be particularly well observed (see Chapter 4, page 36, on the signs of hyperthermia).

The additional buoyancy gained by high body fat content can mean that it is difficult to maintain the vertical position in chest-high water. Balance tends to be poor because there is so little weight through the feet and legs that the normal proprioceptive pathways are not as active. It is necessary to ensure, for safety reasons, that all participants are able to stand and walk safely, and can get from standing to prone or to supine, and from prone to supine and back, in a controlled manner. In other words, that they have static and dynamic postural alignment and control. This will certainly need to be taught to non-swimmers before other activities are commenced, and will need to be checked for with all newcomers. Figure 10.1 illustrates how this is done.

When doing prone or supine exercises, aids to assist flotation will probably not be technically necessary because of the increased buoyancy. However, tangible supports such as floats are of great psychological comfort to those people who are nervous in water. They may require help, or special coaching, to get the floats in the correct place.

Aerobic exercise involves running and perhaps jumping, both activities likely to be unfamiliar to the participants. It is important to teach the correct technique, particularly with regard to the calf. Each step should involve a push-off, so that

Figure 10.1   Techniques to maintain balance.

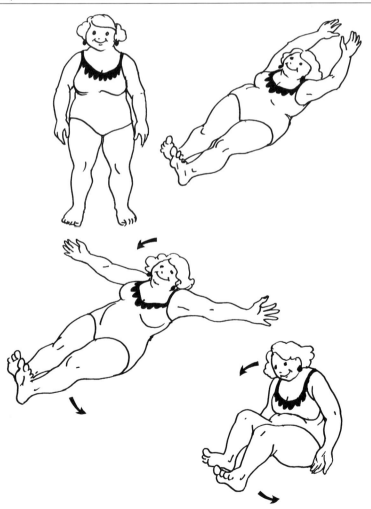

the heels lift up, and the landing, while first onto the toes, continues until the heels are fully lowered onto the floor of the pool. If the heels are not properly replaced, theoretically, this sudden unaccustomed calf use could lead to post-exercise calf soreness. There is also the possibility of causing one of the overuse conditions, such as a tendonitis or bursitis, or a tear to the gastrocnemius or soleus belly or, most seriously, to a rupture of the Achilles tendon. All of these are preventable with correct teaching techniques.

At the end of a vigorous class, it is necessary to drink to prevent dehydration. However, it is good coaching practice to suggest that participants resist the temptation to eat after exercise. It is important, though to encourage a period of rest, by sitting down and having a low calorie drink, or water. An Aquarobics session does not give the right to binge. If in danger of succumbing to 'snacks', then encourage clients to bring an apple or a carrot to nibble afterwards with the drink.

Aims and Objectives of Aquarobics for the Overweight

Although the possibility of losing weight is likely to be the stimulus for participation, there is no guarantee of a successful result. Whether or not weight is lost, overall health and fitness should be enhanced, and a feeling of general well-being (modulated by endorphin release), which might help in complying with an overall calorific reduction programme. (In many cases, over-eating is a depressive manifestation, so mood alteration can be effective intervention.)

Other aims will be the normal fitness aims of improving strength, particularly in the anti-gravity muscles which control the load-bearing joints when not immersed. These are the exten-

sor muscle groups: the quadriceps, the calf, the gluteal and the trunk and head extensors.

Adipose tissue tends to accumulate in certain areas. Theoretically, mobilization of fat in those areas could be increased if the relevant muscles are subjected to mild resistance training. Such localized mobilization of fat is a claim frequently made in the fitness world. No evidence has been found to support this, but it cannot do any harm, and is certainly likely to be psychologically effective. Resistance exercises, using buoyancy as 'weights' should therefore be done for the triceps, the quadriceps and the hamstrings (see Exercises 60, 61, 79, 80 and 81). Abdominal exercises are also essential, not only because the abdomen is usually the greatest reservoir for adipose tissue, but because if the tone in the abdominal muscles, particularly the transversis, can be improved, the waist measurement will be reduced. It is therefore good practice to have a specific strengthening programme for all the abdominal muscles (Exercises 25–40).

The muscles of the pelvic floor have been included in this section, as the additional weight of the abdominal contents puts them at slightly greater risk of dysfunction.

Improved mobility is a fitness objective, and it is certainly good practice to take all joints through a full range of movement during a water workout. Moreover it is good practice to stretch all those muscles which have been strengthened during the course of a session. It will therefore be necessary to stretch the calf, the quadriceps, the hamstrings and the triceps. It is not easy to stretch the abdominals.

Table 10.1 suggest some exercises for the overweight and indicates the underlying rationale. People who are overweight do not need specific, different exercises, however, as almost anything can be adapted. Although the idea of holding

Table 10.1
Suggested exercises for the overweight

Objective	Exercise	Notes	Exercise no.
To check for postural safety and balance	Teach static and dynamic posture and alignment	New participants must be 'water safe'	
To warm-up	Changes		1
	Diagonal arm reaches		2
	Shoulder circling		42, 47
	Shovelling		6
	Leg swinging variations		70, 83
	Walking sideways with lunges		93
	Running on the spot		
To prevent calf injury	Calf stretch		101
To improve aerobic function and assist in weight loss	Running, knees up high with variable arms and legs	Selection depends on level of fitness (see Chapter 11)	
	Jumps, with variable arms and legs	Depending on fitness (see Chapter 11)	
	Spotty dogs	Harder without the jump This is also a strength exercise	
To improve muscular strength and endurance	Progressive sequence		
Abdominals:	Cycling	ALWAYS ensure that the	25
	Toe-out curls	tummy is pulled in to work	26
1. Rectus abdominus	Alternate toe-out curls	the transversis	27
	Sit-scissors		29
	Pancake tucks		30
	Prone body tucks		31
2. Obliques	Helicopters		34
	Twists		35
	U-tucks		38
	Parts and crossovers		39
	Paddle corkscrew		37
	V-shapes		40
Quadriceps	8 o'clock knee bends		72
	One-legged squats	Modified to one leg	85
	Cossackski's		89
	Step-ups		77
	Quadriceps pump		81
	Straight leg swinging		70
	Steam engine circles		65
	Flipper walk		98

Table 10.1 (continued)

Objective	Exercise	Notes	Exercise no.
Hamstrings	Super-glue exercise		73
	Running		96
	Flipper running		98
	Hamstring curl		79
	Hamstring pump		80
	Steam engine circles		65
	Flipper helicopters	Helicopter with flippers	34
Arm work	Biceps–triceps curls		55
	Triceps pump		60
	Resisted arm swinging	Wear flippers/mitts	54
	Wall pushes		68
	Triceps lift		61
Pelvic floor	Pelvic floor contractions		111
To improve flexibility		If cool water, the joint stretches may have to be spread throughout the session	
Muscles	Calf stretch	Muscle stretches for those	101
	Hamstring stretch	groups which have been	102
	Quadriceps stretch	strengthened	103
	Triceps stretch		
Joints	Belly dance	Slow full range joint	11
	Horizontal two-armed eights	mobility exercises	4
	The figurehead		16
	Wall squats		17
	Wall knee rises		76
To relax and unwind in a cool-down	Floating	Floating, with or without	111
	Full-body stretches	buoyancy aids can be done	112
		as partner work	113

special classes for those who have excess body mass has many advantages, it is perhaps more likely that such a person will be present in a heterogenous group.

References

Valadian I, Colenam KA, Dwyer JT and Casey VA (1992) Body Mass Index from childhood to middle age: a fifty year follow up. *Am J Clin Nutr* 56(1): 14–18.

Section III
Aquarobics to Promote Health and Fitness

The Allied Dunbar Survey in the UK showed that only 25% of adults partook of regular, fitness-orientated exercise. The majority of people in the population are therefore classified as inactive, thus not meeting the WHO Guidelines of the quantity of exercise that is conducive to health promotion. The World Health Organization (WHO) Charter states that 'Health is a state of complete physical, mental and social well-being and not merely the absence of disease or infirmity. There is strong evidence that regular physical activity provides people of all ages with substantial health gains that are physical, mental and social and contribute significantly to increased quality of life.'

For the potential health benefits of regular exercise to be maximized, what matters is not how exercise is taken, but how long it lasts, how often and at what intensity, and also to what extent *all* components of fitness are incorporated into the regime.

To be truly effective, each component of an exercise schedule needs to be targeted to a specific tissue. Aerobic function is improved by training the cardiopulmonaryvascular system; muscle function is improved by training for an increase in strength, muscular endurance or power; tissues are mobilized by being subjected to a gentle, meaningful stretch. Chapter 2 gives details of the internationally accepted structure for exercise sessions, namely, the general warm-up / preparation for all tissues, different periods with tissue-specific aims and finally a cool-down to return the body gradually to the pre-exercise state.

Section III looks at specific Aquarobics exercises designed to improve the performance of the cardiovascular and musculoskeletal systems. It is hoped that the resultant improvement in physical parameters will also bring about a feeling of enhanced well-being. It is generally recognized that people feel better after participating in appropriate exercise (even if they are not always enjoying it at the time). Intense exercise liberates endorphins, which are similar in function to the opiates, acting as mood-lifters and analgesics. LIke opiates (although to a much lesser degree), they have addictive qualities which may perhaps help to encourage the continuation of regular intense exercise. There is a risk, though, that long-term sustained exercise, such as long-distance running, can in itself become an addictive activity.

So now all the physiological components come together. This section will look at the cardiovascular, muscular strength and endurance, and flexibility aspects of aquatic exercise, in the hope that the whole will promote a feeling of enhanced well-being and fitness, enrich the life of the participants and promote health.

11

Aerobic Training

It will be remembered from Chapter 2, on exercise physiology, that marked adaptations to the cardiovascular system occur on immersion. To summarize, hydrostatic pressure on the lower body causes a shift of blood and interstitial fluid of about 700 ml to the central cavity. This increases the stroke volume, and results in a reduction of about 10 beats per minute to the resting heart rate. The exact amount of fluid that shifts centrally will depend on the individual, the depth of immersion and, to a minor extent, the temperature of the water. The studies on which this data was based were performed with the subjects at rest, and seated to the level of the xiphisternum.

If the main objective of an exercise is to improve cardiorespiratory function then, what do we mean by this?, how do we know it is happening?, and what are the pros and cons of doing this in the water as compared to dry-land cardiovascular training?

The parameters which indicate an improvement in the function of the cardiovascular system include the resting heart rate and the time that the heart takes to return to its resting rate after exertion, both of which should reduce with cardiovascular training. The best objective index of the efficiency of the cardiovascular system and the lungs is a measurement of VO_2 max, (see Chapter 2) but this is difficult to do in a labora-tory or gymnasium setting, let alone in a swimming pool where it is not only difficult to collect expired gases as the subject works towards exhaustion, but almost impossible to quantify the amount of work done. The Borg Scale of Perceived Effort gives a useful subjective measure, and can be combined with a measurement of the heart rate, and the changes in rate as effort increases and decreases.

Does Aquatic Exercise Produce an Aerobic Training Effect?

Despite the practical difficulties, several studies have compared the results of undertaking aerobic training programmes performed on dry land and in water. Three studies used cycle ergometry as the form of exercise. Avellini et al. (1983) compared three groups of unconditioned young men who were trained for one month, using cycle ergometry. One group was not immersed. The other groups did their exercise in water at either 32 °C or 20 °C. All groups demonstrated improvement in VO_2 max, despite a significantly lower heart rate in the cold water group. Sheldahl et al. (1986) found that both land and water groups had similar increases in stroke volume and decreases in heart rate and blood pressure, when compared to the inactive controls. Christie et al.

(1990) found similar VO_2 max at different work intensities on land and when immersed. This study involved internal cardiac catheters and so was able to compare many different cardiac parameters. Heart rates were significantly lower ($P < 0.05$) in water only during the two highest work intensities (80% and 100% maximal).

Svedenhag and Seger (1992) compared ten trained runners at different target heart rates including maximal heart rate when immersed and on a treadmill. For a given volume of oxygen consumed per minute, the heart rate was 8–11 beats lower when immersed, but perceived exertion and respiratory exchange were higher. They concluded that 'immersion induces acute cardiac adjustments that extend up to the maximal exercise level.'

It appears that the temperature of the water affects the cardiac adjustments. This was implied in Avellini's study quoted above, and observed by Hall *et al.* (1998) who demonstrated that heart rate was higher during chest-deep water walking in water at 36 °C (115 beats/min) than on a land treadmill (106 beats/min) or in water at 28 °C (99.6 beats/min). Furthermore Kirby *et al.* (1984), who were concerned about the potential risk of exercising in a heated hydrotherapy pool at 36 °C. They concluded that vigorous exercises in such a pool not only stresses aerobic capacity in normal individuals, but could be a risk to post-myocardial infarct patients.

A study by Cassady and Nielson (1992) evaluated the oxygen consumption and heart rate response curves for standardized upper and lower extremity exercise on land and in water, in 40 healthy subjects. The oxygen consumption and heart rate increased as the exercise intensity was increased. The former was higher in the water but the percentage of age-predicted maximal heart rate was greater during land exercise. This is consistent with the above studies.

The Advantages of Aquatic Exercise

The advantage of training whilst immersed is that the buoyancy of water reduces the risk of injury, and therefore allows some people to partake in an aerobic training programme, for whom it would be painful or difficult to do so on dry land. However, for training to be safe, certain procedures must be observed. Firstly, there must be a gradual warm-up period, during which time the heart rate is raised. This is not to be confused with the warm-up which happens at the beginning of the class. This second 'warm-up' period is sometimes referred as the 'pulse raiser'. Secondly, the aerobic training period should last for long enough to achieve the training effect. This is dependent on the intensity of training. Similar increases in cardiorespiratory endurance may be achieved by a low intensity, long duration session as well as by a higher intensity, shorter duration session. ACSM recommends that the intensity of exercise be prescribed as 60 to 90% of maximum heart rate, or 50–85% of VO_2 max. Finally, the training heart rate should be reduced over a period of two or three minutes, and not suddenly lowered by stopping or standing still. This latter could cause a sudden fall in blood pressure which could be hazardous. Figure 11.1 shows the aerobic training curve for cardiovascular function.

The heart muscle is wonderfully responsive to need and will only work just hard enough to supply oxygen-rich blood to the demanding muscles and other tissues, and remove the 'debris' of metabolism. If the demand drops, then the heart rate will reduce quickly.

There are two factors which theoretically put additional load on to this pumping system, when the exercise is taking place standing up in water.

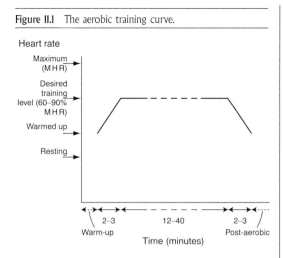

Figure II.I   The aerobic training curve.

from any dry-land target that is calculated.

The heart rate cannot be measured manually during exercise, as the rate will have dropped significantly by the time the carotid or wrist pulse has been located. The only accurate means of knowing whether cardiovascular training is taking place is to use waterproof cardiac monitors which give an average heart rate reading with samples taken at variable but frequent intervals. However, after a few weeks of regular training, it is hoped that the dry-land benefits should be obvious to the participant by observations such as being able to run upstairs, or to catch a bus, without getting as 'puffed out' as before.

The first is that the kidneys continue to require blood even though exercise is taking place. (The antidiuretic hormone, which normally reduces kidney activity when exercising on dry land, does not function in the same way when immersed, see Chapter 2.) The second relates to temperature: the heart may be affected if the pool is either too cold or too warm. A warm pool causes vasodilation, which places an additional demand on the heart as blood is not then being shunted away from the skin to be diverted to the demanding working muscles. A very cold pool might cause vasoconstriction with an accompanying increase in blood pressure. These comments, however, relate to extremes in temperature, i.e. above 30 °C and below 20 °C.

The most important fact to remember is that the heart rate when *sitting* at rest, immersed, is about 10 beats per minute below that when not immersed. Ideally, aerobic training should be done standing in chest-high water, which will theoretically decrease the heart rate even further than 10 beats a minute, because the hydrostatic pressure on the feet and legs is greater when standing than when sitting. The target heart rates should therefore be reduced by ten beats per minute

Techniques for Raising the Heart Rate Into a Training Zone

In the water (unless there is rapid displacement of large volumes of water), there is much less effort involved in movement than when doing the same exercise non-immersed. In order to increase the heart rate, therefore, it is necessary to work many major muscle groups at the same time, and work them hard and fast. There is increased loading on the heart when the arms are above the head, but it is not necessary to keep them in that position for too long, as hard pulling and pushing moves that displace water are also movements that involve many muscle groups working hard.

The important factors to bear in mind when increasing the workload on the heart doing vertical exercise are the speed of the movement, the shape of the moving part, the length of the lever and where the arms are in relation to the heart. Large-scale fast movements are usually necessary.

Table II.I gives an example of a progressive sequence, which will gradually increase the load

Table 11.1
Progression of aerobic activities, from easier to harder

Activity	Limb movements	Speed	Other factors
Running on the spot	Short lever, i.e. flexed knees and elbows. Shoulder and hip movements getting larger	Start slow and get faster. Punch the water surface to make 'white water'	Vary the direction; not always facing front, but turning and twisting
Running around the pool. Need to change direction often, or it gets easier	Always opposite arm and leg together. Get a good push off with the toes. Aim for large-scale movements	Impossible to do too fast. Can be team games or aerobic circuit, but keep them moving	Vary arm and leg moves. Make formations, e.g. vary directions: inner and outer circles going different ways
Moving on the spot	Long levers; straight knees and elbows. Position the hands and fingers to make maximum resistance	The additional lever length means you have to slow down a little; it is hard work. Vary the activities	The water should be chest-high to prevent too much impact
Total body moves (see Aerobic exercises, Section IV)	These are complex movement patterns; some are stationary, others move around	Should be done as fast as possible	
Jumps	Most jumps involve specific arm and leg positions	Slow down a little, to allow enough time for correct technique, and the recovery of balance	Stress the importance of taking off and landing correctly

on the CV system. The classic sign of correct working within the aerobic training zone is breathlessness without distress. Once clients are warmed-up, and have been screened and warned about the purpose of the exercise that they are about to do, the aquatic coach will start doing the 'pulse-raising,' easy activities shown at the top of Table 11.1. To improve aerobic function, it is necessary to hold the intensity of peak activity for any individual at that level which would render them breathless, but still able to carry out a conversation. This level is then held for the required time (minimum 12 minutes, maximum 35 minutes), before being slowly reduced. The degree of breathlessness would indicate whether the train-

ing was at 60% or 70% of the calculated maximum heart rate.

The appropriate entry point for any individual will depend on their fitness level. Obviously somebody who is totally unaccustomed to exercise, and perhaps elderly, would 'peak' at a much lower level than an athlete. Indeed, while this range of aerobic demand might be geared too high for the former individual, who could be getting breathless simply walking around the pool, the range could be too low for really aerobically fit individuals, who may need to don buoyancy supports and run in deep water to get sufficiently breathless.

Table 11.1 can be used in conjunction with Section IV, Part G to select specific exercises which will demonstrate a progression of aerobic activities, from easier to harder. After the 'peak' intensity has been maintained for the requisite time, the level should be reduced somewhat, so as to return the aerobic curve to the level before the 'pulse raiser'.

References

Avellini BA, Shapiro Y and Pandolf KB (1983) Cardio-respiratory physical training in water and on land. *Eur J Appl Physiol* **50**: 255–263.

Cassady SL and Nielson DH (1992) Cardiorespiratory responses of healthy subjects to calisthenics performed on land versus in water. *Phys Ther* **72**: 5532–5538.

Christie JL, Sheldahl LM, Tristant FE *et al.* (1990) Cardiovascular regulation during head-out water immersion exercise. *J Appl Physiol* **69**(2): 657–664.

Hall J, Macdonald IA, Maddison PJ and O'Hare JP (1998) Cardiorespiratory responses to underwater treadmill walking in healthy females. *Eur J Appl Physiol* **77**: 278–284.

Kirby RL, Sacamano JT, Balch DE and Kriellaars DJ (1984) Oxygen consumption during exercise in a heated pool. *Arch Phys Med Rehabil* **65**: 21–23.

Sheldahl LM, Tristani FE, Clifford PS *et al.* (1986) Effect of head-out water immersion on response to exercise training. *Appl Physiol* **60**(6): 1878–1881.

Svedenhag J and Seger J (1992) Running on land and in water. Comparative exercise physiology. *Med Sci Sports Exerc* **24**(10): 1155–1160.

World Health Organization (1997) *WHO Meeting Stresses Health Benefits of 'Active Living'.* Press Release/19. WHO, Geneva.

12

Enhancing Muscle Function

Participating in fitness activities, such as going to a gym and carrying out systematic resistance and aerobic training is one of the fastest growing leisure pursuits. Health Clubs and Leisure Centres are proliferating, and are being utilized by happy exercisers, of all ages, sizes and shapes. Even though the majority of the population is still sedentary (Allied Dunbar, 1994) the substantial increase in the number of people wanting to undertake exercises to improve their overall fitness implies that they feel they are deriving benefit from such activity.

Resistance Training

The beneficial effects of taking part in a resistance training programme go beyond strengthening the actual muscles that are being exercised. As well as the increases in the size of individual fibres and the overall muscle mass, the enhancement in performance, and the improvement in many biochemical parameters, there is also an increase in bone density and a feeling of well-being. Resistance training is probably the best and simplest antidote to osteoporosis, and it is never too late to start (Beverley *et al.*, 1989; Skelton *et al.*, 1995).

Strength

Normally, resistance training involves working a particular muscle (or group) through its full range, at a slow steady speed, so that there is a substantial load on the muscle(s) throughout the range. Usually the load selected is such that the movement can only be performed 10–20 times before fatigue sets in. Now, all of this refers to a dry-land situation, and it does not matter whether the load is body weight, free or fixed weights, or specialized gym machinery. It is extremely difficult, if not impossible, to perform the same exercises in the water, and achieve the same results, but nonetheless some enhancement of muscle function can be obtained, although probably not an increase in strength as measured by the once-only maximal lift.

The reason for the difference is because 'weights' do not weigh the same when immersed, and it is therefore usually not possible to produce a load that will tire the muscles in only 10–20 repetitions when exercising aquatically. However, as well as strength, there are two other aspects to muscle performance, endurance and power, and both of these can be improved by appropriate aquatic exercise, possibly more easily and effectively than in a gym. Moreover, as muscle work in water is concentric, the process of carrying out any full range movement is likely to work both agonists and antagonists equally, thereby producing a more balanced work-out, and one without risk of the post-exercise soreness caused by eccentric contraction. Any subsequent anthropomorphic changes will therefore apply equally to all muscle groups exercised, and therefore not interfere with range. (Excessive dry land work such as 'Step' can cause such increase in the bulk of the quadriceps that the hamstring length becomes compromised.)

Power and Endurance

Resistance training in the pool is therefore geared towards power and endurance work. Power is a combination of strength and speed. It is still necessary to work the muscle against a load, and to carry out a full range movement. To improve power and endurance, perform full-range exercises to individual muscle or muscle groups, so that fatigue is caused, preferably after 30–40 fast repetitions. The easiest way to increase the load in the pool is to increase the speed of the movement, the length of the lever, and the resistance through the water, by forming an unstreamlined posture with the moving part. Each of these points will be dealt with separately.

SPEED OF MOVEMENT

Assuming that any movement is through as large a range as possible, the faster that this happens, the more turbulence is created, the greater the effort to move through that turbulence and hence, the greater the torque on the working muscles. A common mistake is to reduce the range of movement as the speed of movement increases. It might seem difficult to work-to-fatigue to music, which may have the wrong rhythm to facilitate maximal effort. There is a little trick that solves this problem: it is known as 'the whoosh'! Clients are instructed to move as fast as they can through the water, in as large a movement as possible – in one direction only, on the 'down-beat', whilst thinking of making a 'whooshing' through the water. There is then a brief pause before returning to the starting position on the next down-beat. This is a way of working as fast as possible, but still using the rhythm of the music to provide a framework.

LEVER LENGTH

It is obviously easier to produce a long lever when exercising the hip and shoulder, than when exercising the knee or elbow, as all that is necessary is to hold those intermediate joints in an extended position. It is therefore easy to improve power and endurance in the hip or shoulder (or indeed both at the same time, by performing reciprocal limb swinging exercises). In order to build up similar torques in the muscles acting on the knee and elbow joints, the wrist and fingers can be held in a straight position, or a flipper can be worn on the hand or foot.

RESISTANCE THROUGH THE WATER

The resistance, and hence the load, can be increased by adopting unstreamlined postures, by wearing webbed gloves or flippers, or holding unstreamlined objects such as floats, Frisbees, etc. The resistance will be reduced if the movement facilitates the formation of circular eddy currents, so circular movements must be avoided.

Using Floats: The Buoyancy Effect

In the above considerations, resistance and turbulence have been the property of water that has affected the effort of movement. By using buoyant objects, such as floats, buoyancy can also be used to increase effort. In order to be most effective, the effort must go into pushing the float vertically downwards. The problem is that the muscle work, instead of always being concentric, will change so that it is concentric when pushing downwards, but eccentric when moving vertically upwards (see Chapter 3). This is, of course, opposite to dry-land exercise when muscle work is concentric when going upwards and eccentric when going downwards. It must also be remembered that there is more possibility of post-exercise pain because of the eccentric muscle work.

References

Allied Dunbar (1994) A report on activity patterns and fitness levels. London Health Education Authority/Sports Council.

American College of Sports Medicine (ACSM) (1995) *Guidelines for Exercise Testing and Prescription*, 5th edn. Williams & Wilkins, Baltimore.

Beverley MC, Rider TA, Evans MJ and Smith R (1989) Local bone mineral response to brief exercise that stresses the skeleton. *Br Med J* **299**: 233–235.

Skelton DA, Young A, Greig CA and Malbut KE (1995) Effects of resistance training on strength, power and selected functional abilities of women aged 75 and older. *J Am Geriatr Soc* **43**(10): 1081–1087.

13

Improving Flexibility

One might say, with tongue in cheek, that life, from the moment of birth, is a gradual process of stiffening up – until the final rigidity of death. Certainly young children are much more flexible than adults, but this is largely due to the fact that the skeleton is still somewhat pliable. It is, however, not just bone, or even bone and joint tissues which determine the flexibility of any individual. Restrictions or adhesions in connective tissue including skin, muscle, ligaments and even neural tissue can all cause localized or widespread loss of flexibility. In fact, it is probable that even without damage to such tissues, simply not stretching out to the normal range of movement will eventually result in a reduction in that so-called 'normal' range. The body could be looked on like one of those early forms of plastic – originally mouldable and flexible but eventually brittle and self-destructible.

Many of the arthritic conditions that can lead to lack of flexibility are precipitated by damaged joints (see Chapter 8). Such syndromes are often extremely painful and disabling and can interfere seriously with lifestyle. This chapter, though, is not concerned with specific diseases, but with ranges of so-called normal flexibility, and how to maintain and increase them. It will examine the factors concerned with the maintenance of flexi-

bility and how this may be improved by aquatic exercise. It will discuss the difficulties of performing flexibility exercises in water, both as regards getting the necessary force to 'stretch' the desired tissues and with maintaining core body temperature whilst carrying out such exercises.

Structures Involved in Flexibility

As stated earlier, the degree of flexibility in any individual is, to some extent, dependent on age. It will now be assumed that we are dealing only with adults whose skeletons are fully developed. How can the flexibility of early adult life be maintained? Each of the important tissues which affect overall flexibility will be looked at in relation to aquatic exercise.

Skin

Skin is a structure which is normally fairly pliable, and does not become contracted without disease process, or trauma such as burning. It is therefore largely irrelevant as regards aquatic exercise.

Muscles

Current practice dictates that muscles should be stretched before and after exercise. This is said to be done for two reasons: firstly it is said to reduce the incidence of muscle injuries and secondly, it is purported to reduce post-exercise muscle pain. This latter phenomenon is more likely if the muscles concerned have been challenged eccentrically, rather than concentrically. Unless floats are used, muscle work when immersed is concentric. Newham (1988) found that post-exercise muscle soreness is primarily a phenomenon of eccentric contractions, and is therefore unlikely to follow an aquatic work-out, which is primarily concentric.

In order to stretch effectively, the joints upon which the muscle acts need to be correctly positioned. This will, of course, vary with each muscle, but postures for the common muscles are discussed briefly below, and in more detail in Part H of Section IV, on Flexibility.

Whenever muscles are stretched it must be done in a slow, steady way, being held for about 20 seconds. If the stretches become fast and bouncy, they risk triggering the muscle stretch reflex, which could result in a contraction (and possible tear) of the muscle fibres. It is obviously more effective to stretch a relaxed muscle, rather than fight any contraction. There are two active ways to increase muscle relaxation. If the desired muscle is strongly contracted against resistance, then a deeper degree of relaxation will probably follow. A more effective method is to contract the antagonist muscle. Thus, if wanting to stretch the hamstrings, one would first contract the quadriceps against resistance, and then stretch the hamstrings. This technique is known as *proprioceptive neuromuscular facilitation* (PNF).

The purpose of pre-exercise stretching is reputed to be the prevention of injury, although there is a dearth of literature confirming the claim. Even accepting that this prophylaxis is effective, pre-exercise stretching need only take a short time,

about 15–20 seconds per muscle, and needs to concentrate on those muscles most at risk. In the water, the muscle which is most at risk is the calf, because aquatic exercises like jumping are not usually performed in dry-land classes. It is important that all clients are taught that the heels should be replaced on the pool floor between each step or jump. If not, the entire class could be done in the tip-toes position, and this, added to the unaccustomed jumping could well result in, at best, post-exercise soreness, and at worst injury to the calf muscle or the Achilles tendon. Because muscle stretching is a comparatively static activity, standing still can result in rapid heat loss. This counteracts all the good effect of the warm-up which should already have happened. It is therefore advisable to keep pre-exercise stretching to a bare minimum.

During a dry land exercise session, there is often an extended stretching session at the end. Such stretches are known more as 'developmental stretches'. These are held for longer than the pre-exercise stretching (20 seconds to one minute) and the stretch is increased as the body adjusts to the stretching sensation. It is after exercise, when the body is fully warmed up, that extra flexibility is gained, but this needs to be done slowly and carefully, lest injury to muscle fibre result. It is not always possible to stretch as effectively in the water, as there is not the body weight to push against the stretched position. There is also the real risk of becoming cold.

Joints

Every joint has its natural range of movement, which needs to be taken to those natural limits fairly often. If a perfectly healthy joint is encapsulated in plaster, through injury to an adjoining area, then that joint will be extremely stiff when the plaster is removed. In Chapter 8 on arthritis, it is seen that degenerative changes can happen after injury or forced immobilization.

Neural Tissue

The significance of maintaining normal flexibility in nerve tissue has really only been appreciated in the past few years. It has been known for centuries that a pain in the distribution of the sciatic nerve as a result of having one straight leg passively raised — a positive SLR test (see Glossary) — is the classic sign of a low lumbar disc lesion. An SLR test is illustrated in Figure 13.1. Tissue, probably from the prolapsed disc, takes up space within the neural canal, and restricts the passive stretch which needs to occur as the leg is lifted. If the head and the leg are lifted at the same time, the distance from the toes to the brain is increased, thereby increasing the stretch and the likelihood of producing pain.

It is now known that normal flexibility demands that not only the spinal cord, but all neural tissue, be free to glide within their surrounding membranes. Any restriction, such as that caused by trauma which leads to microscopic bleeding and the formation of scar tissue, can reduce this vital neural flexibility by tying down the nerves within their sheaths. In the long term this is a major predisposing factor to spinal pain. There are certain anchorage points throughout the body, but elsewhere neural tissue needs to be able to move freely within its protective membranes. It is now believed that positive neural tension signs (see Glossary) contribute to all sorts of diverse mechanical musculoskeletal conditions, from tennis elbow to plantar fasciitis.

Figure 13.1   Straight leg raise test.

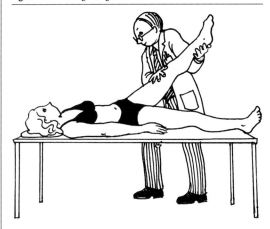

Practical Considerations

It has been seen that there are many aspects to the improvement in flexibility. Doing stretching in water has advantages and disadvantages over doing them on dry land. In the water there is the real risk of getting cold — and this is counterproductive for several reasons, one of which is that it is always better to stretch warm tissues. An advantage of aquatic flexibility is that certain dynamic stretching exercises, such as the Pike, can be done, which would be impossible elsewhere.

The flexibility exercises can be found in Section IV, Part H. They are subdivided by body part and by type of stretch.

Reference

Newham DJ (1988) The consequences of eccentric contraction and their relationship to delayed onset muscle pain. *Eur J Appl Physiol* 57(3): 353–359.

Section IV
The Exercises

Total Body Movement

·

Spinal Exercises

·

Abdominals Exercises

·

Upper Quadrant

·

Lower Quadrant

·

Locomotion Exercises

·

Balance Exercises

·

Aerobic Combinations

·

Flexibility

·

Pelvic Floor

·

Relaxation

It is hoped that this section will be the key reference part of the book, and it has been arranged to make this as easy as possible. Not only are the purposes and uses of each individual exercise given clearly, but they have been arranged by body part and overall function.

As the spine can be looked on as the link to all other body parts, this has been placed next after the 'Total body' section. Because most exercises in water are not confined to a single joint, but are more regional, the spine has been divided into upper and lower regions. Whereas many of the upper spinal exercises will also work the arms and shoulder girdle, the lower spinal exercises also involve the hip joints, and sometimes the knees. This regional emphasis reflects the way in which the body works when doing normal functional activities.

The exercises are subdivided into groups. These groups relate to part of the body, and to the reason for doing the exercise. The body has been divided into six regions, the upper and lower spine and the abdominal muscles, the upper and lower quadrants (i.e. the respective limb and relating part of the torso) and the pelvic floor. To assist with finding suitable exercises for rehabilitation, there are a further two categories to cover locomotion exercises and balance training.

Finally, the entire list of exercises has been assembled, more or less in the order in which one might come to them chronologically if doing an aquatic work-out. In other words, there are warm-up exercises first, then muscle work. This is followed by a separate classification for exercises which are designed to work the body aerobically, and finally, there are the cool-down and flexibility exercises, culminating with relaxation. If more than one exercise achieves the same purpose, they are classified according to the degree of effort, from easy to harder. The exercises have been described, as far as possible, in a non-medical way. This is not only because fitness coaches are not as accustomed to medical and anatomical jargon as are physiotherapists, but because the actual words used may be useful in the teaching process to patients and clients. They have been developed over many years of practical pool experience, as an easy way to communicate movement with patients. A Summary Table of Exercises is given here for quick reference.

No indication is given of how many times each exercise should be performed, as this depends on so many different factors. The skilled physiotherapist and fitness coach will know instinctively when to move on to a different exercise.

To make the description of the exercises easier to follow, it is assumed that all unilateral exercises will be repeated on the opposite side. This may involve turning round and facing the other way.

It has not been easy to compile these exercises in a logical sequence, because the uses are so diverse and the starting points so variable. What would be a tough warm-up exercise for one person could be the peak aerobic activity for another. The same exercise could even improve muscle performance, by increasing strength and/or endurance in yet a third individual. Everybody is an individual, and will have a different starting point.

In some ways, this is the crux of Aquarobics. A successful practitioner will not be routinely following exercises, as a cook follows menus. They will adapt and create as they proceed. The enclosed exercises can therefore be looked on as mere sketches, leaving the physiotherapist or the aquatic coach space to put in the colours and complete the picture.

List of exercises

A TOTAL BODY MOVEMENT

This exercise is a very useful way of starting Aquarobics sessions, regardless of fitness level or pathology present. It allows time for the clients to make the necessary proprioceptive adjustments in order to keep their balance in the water, as well as time for introduction and explanation, all of which can happen whilst this useful exercise is being performed. It is called 'The Changes', because body weight is being changed from foot to foot.

I. THE CHANGES

Why do it?

To get the feeling of moving in the water. To mobilize the ankles, toes, knees and spine. To restore the bounce to walking. To develop coordination between the arms and the legs, by mimicking jogging arm movement. To get warm, especially if the water is cold; and establish a repetitive functional movement, which can be continued whilst giving and receiving information, e.g. screening and explaining the principles. To begin to increase the load on the cardiovascular system.

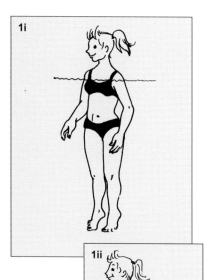

Starting position

Stand with the feet just a little apart. Unaccustomed, or overweight exercisers may need to start at (a). Most people will be able to go straight to (b).

Movement

(a) To begin with, go up and down on your toes, so that both feet bend at the big toe joints, but the knees are straight (1i).

(b) When you are comfortable doing that without feeling that you are falling over, then transfer your weight from one foot to the other, by peeling one heel off the floor of the pool (with the other foot flat), but leaving the big toe in contact with the floor of the pool. As each heel rises in turn, so the knee of the leg that is lifting up will bend forward. Throughout this sequence you will need to imagine that each big toe is stuck to the floor of the pool (1ii).

(c) Finally, continue pumping the weight from one big toe to the other, but getting a feeling of bounce as you do it. The head should bob up and down with each step. This is a stationary exercise.

Progressions

1.   Keep the elbows still and swing the arms in a reciprocal motion to the legs (i.e. right arm and left leg are forward together; 1ii).

2.   Make the arm movement harder by positioning the hands and fingers to increase the resistance when moving through the water.

3.   Twist the upper and lower body more, so that the knee is more or less directly under the opposite elbow, thereby increasing spinal rotation (see 'Changes with Exaggerated Limbs', page 145).

B SPINAL EXERCISES

Upper spine

The following eight exercises are primarily for mobility. They can be used as warm-up exercises in the absence of local pathology. The normal reciprocal limb walking pattern involves spinal rotation. This rotation can be clearly observed from the rear in somebody walking whilst swinging their arms. As this seems the most natural and normal of functional movements – this spinal rotation is used first in any exercise session – spinal flexion, extension and side flexion will follow later.

2. DIAGONAL ARM REACHES

Why do it?

To start to rotate the lower spine – perhaps the most functional activity as it is necessary for walking. To mobilize the shoulder complex. To assist in weight transference by doing a lunge motion.

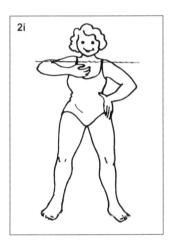
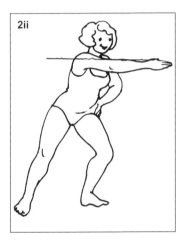
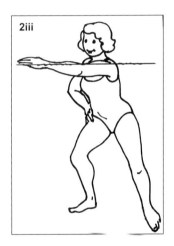

Starting position

Stand in chest-high water, with the feet shoulder-width apart.

Movement

(a) **The arms:** place the left hand on the left hip and reach diagonally with the right hand across the front of your body, towards the left (2i).

(b) **The legs:** As you reach over towards the left, transfer your weight mostly onto the left knee, which you bend. The right knee stays straight (2ii).

(c) Return to the starting position and repeat to the other side (2iii). Continue reaching (and lunging) to alternate sides.

Teaching points

1. In order to avoid twisting the knee, make sure that the bent knee is always directly over the foot.

2. In a class situation, this is very effective as a formation. Two lines of people face each other, a short way apart, so that the 'reaching' hands can touch.

Progression

Diagonal arm reaches with 'extensions': As one hand reaches across the front of the body, the other hand reaches behind the body, thereby increasing the amount of rotation. All the weight can be transferred onto the lunging leg, so that the other leg is lifted out to enhance the diagonal.

3. BASIC CORKSCREW

Why do it?

To mobilize the thoracic spine and rib cage. To work the trunk muscles and to facilitate balance.

Starting position

Stand, preferably in chest-high water, with the feet shoulder-width apart, and the arms floating on the surface with the elbows flexed to about 90 degrees (3i).

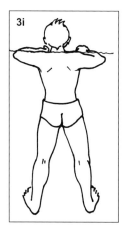

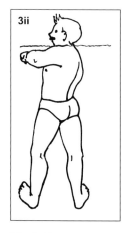

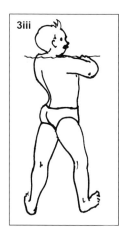

Movement

Rotate from the hips so that the entire upper body and head turn round to one side (3ii), then reverse direction to go the other way (3iii).

Variations

Localize the movement to just spine, or spine and hips by squeezing the buttocks so as to fix them.

---

4. HORIZONTAL TWO-ARMED EIGHTS

Why do it?

To warm up the upper trunk and arms, and to start gentle rotation.

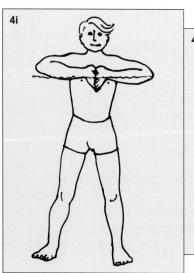

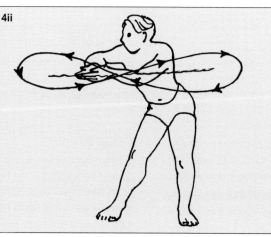

Starting position

Stand with the feet apart and the hands held to the front with the elbows at right angles and the palms facing each other (4i).

Movement

Keeping the palms in the same relative positions, move both forearms and trunk (rotating from the waist) so that they make a large figure-of-eight to your front and sides (4ii).

5. SIDE BENDS

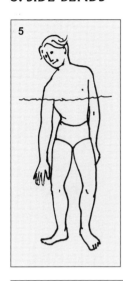

Why do it?

To work the trunk muscles, especially the side-flexors. To provide an initial mobilization for the facet, sacro-iliac and hip joints in a warm-up situation.

Starting position

Stand with the feet about shoulder-width apart.

Movement

Keeping the elbows straight, push down to one side, so as to bend at the waist. See how far you can reach down the outside of your leg. Repeat to the opposite side, either alternately, or after a 'set' of about 16.

Teaching points

Try to keep the centre of gravity central, in other words, discourage the hips being pushed from side to side.

---

6. SHOVELLING

This exercise is difficult to describe. It is similar to a whole body shovelling movement, and involves moving diagonally, with one foot leading, with a shuffle step.

Why do it?

This is an active whole body exercise.

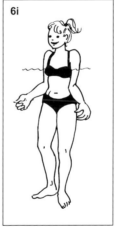

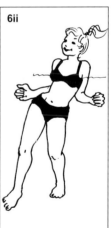

Starting position

Stand with the feet touching, so that the right foot is in front, points diagonally forwards and outwards and the right heel is touching the instep of the left foot. Place the arms as though shovelling, with the elbows tucked into the waist (6i).

Movement

(a) Step diagonally forward with the right leg, swaying from the hips so that they stick out behind. At the same time, 'shovel' with the arms (6ii).

(b) Follow with the left foot, so that it returns to its original alignment touching the right heel. As you move forward exaggerate the pelvic thrust and continue to make a 'shovelling' movement with the arms and upper trunk moving in one piece.

(c) Repeat moving two or three steps in the same direction.

(d) Lead with the left foot and zig-zag to the next diagonal, reversing the feet.

(e) Turn round to get back to the starting position. It does not work well going backwards.

7. MUSCLE MAN ARM CYCLING

Why do it?

To mobilize the shoulder and arm joints.

Starting position

(a) Adopt the position that a 'body-builder' would take up, if he were displaying his right biceps with his left arm bent behind (7i).

(b) Turn the shoulders to the right, and keep the head and feet stationary throughout (7ii).

Movement

Turn the body to the right, while reversing the position of right and left arms (7iii). You will find that the elbows have gone through a cycling motion. Continue this cycling, alternating between the two arms.

Progression

Wear glove flippers, or hold an unstreamlined, non-buoyant, small object.

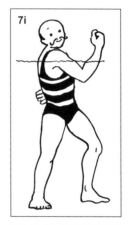

7i

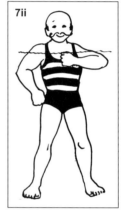

7ii

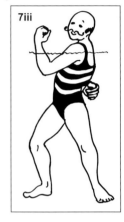

7iii

8. SHOULDER GIRDLE BEND AND STRETCH

Why do it?

To increase flexibility in the arms and shoulders, to help coordination in the muscles of the neck, upper trunk and arms. To strengthen those same muscles.

Starting position

Stand in shoulder-high water with the feet apart and the little fingers touching the front of the shoulders (8i).

Movement

(a) Stretch both arms in front of you, while turning the palms to face outwards as you reach (so that when your arms are fully extended the backs of the hands are touching each other; 8ii). As you do this, the neck shortens and the shoulders rise.

(b) Reverse the movement, turning the palms downwards and inwards as you go, so that the shoulders are pulled back with the elbows bent behind you. The hands should be close to the shoulders.

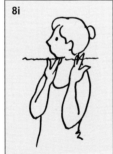

8i

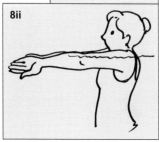

8ii

9. ARM CIRCLE WALKING

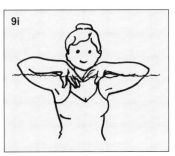

9i

Why do it?

To mobilize the shoulder and scapulae joints. To work many of the muscles around the shoulder complex, and to improve coordination.

Starting position

Stand, with the feet a little way apart, and place the hands so that they are just touching the point of the shoulder on the same side. Make sure that the shoulders are immersed; if necessary, flex the knees (9i).

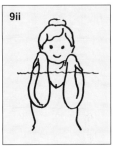

9ii

Movement

(a) Circle the elbows, making as large a movement as possible. Try to get the elbows to touch each other, in the front (9ii).

(b) Walk forwards when the arms circle in a forward direction.

Variations

Circle clockwise and anticlockwise. Have the circles in, or out of synchrony. Vary the direction of the walking to what seems to go naturally with the arms.

Lower Spine

The following exercises are primarily for mobility. They can be used as warm-up exercises, in the absence of local pathology.

EXERCISES THAT ARE PRIMARILY FOR ROTATION

Arranged in increasing order of range of movement and effort.

10. CHANGES WITH EXAGGERATED LIMBS

This is the final progression of the first exercise, 'The Changes'.

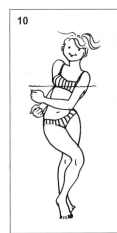

10

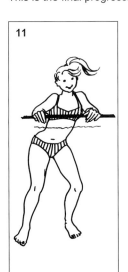

11

11. BELLY DANCE

Why do it?

- To increase flexibility in the lumbar spine.
- To prevent and treat lumbar disc problems.
- To work the abdominal muscles.
- To improve coordination in the pelvic area

Starting position

Stand facing the side of the pool, holding on just far enough away so that the arms and back are straight. The feet should be as wide apart as the hips, so that the legs are vertical. Bend both knees just a little bit, while keeping the back straight. The tummy should be sucked in flat throughout this exercise.

Movement

Rotate the pelvis, as though manipulating a hula-hoop, or doing an Egyptian belly dance.

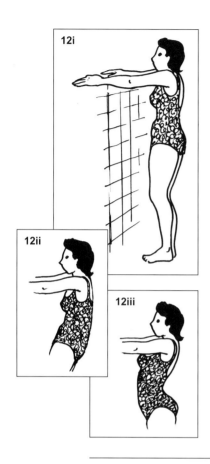

EXERCISES THAT PRIMARILY INVOLVE FLEXION AND EXTENSION

12. BUMPS AND GRINDS

Why do it?

It mobilizes the lumbar spine and pelvis in a natural way.

Starting position

Stand facing the side of the pool, holding on just far enough away so that the arms and back are straight. The feet should be as wide apart as the hips, so that the legs are vertical. Bend both knees just a little bit, while keeping the back straight. The tummy should be sucked in flat throughout this exercise (12i).

Movement

Flatten and arch the lumbar spine (without moving the knees) so that the small of the back is alternately 'humping' (12ii) and 'hollowing' (12iii). Only the pelvis should move, the top half of the body being anchored by the arms. (This movement bears more than a passing resemblance to a striptease artiste in action.)

Teaching point

A common fault is to flex and extend the knees, instead of localizing the movement to the lumbar spine.

13. SQUAT TUCKS

This is similar to the previous exercise, but because it is done in a more flexed position, it is particularly suitable as an antenatal exercise. It is also a more localized spinal exercise, and is therefore slightly harder.

Why do it?

To increase flexion and extension in the lumbar spine, and to assist in spinal stability.

Starting position

Hold on to the side of the pool and place the feet fairly wide apart. Bend the knees as though doing a ballet plié. In other words, keep the trunk vertical and the weight over the heels (not as though sitting in a chair).

Movement

Without moving the knees at all, tuck in your 'tail', so as to flex the lumbar spine. Hold the tuck for the count of 10, then slowly release and repeat.

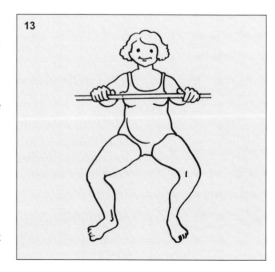

14. KNEES UP

Why do it?

To warm-up the hip flexors and gluteal muscles and mobilize the lower lumbar spine and hips.

Starting position

Stand with the feet together. Hold on with one hand, if necessary.

Movement

(a) Flex one hip and knee as high as possible.

(b) Allow the head and shoulders to relax forwards a little, so as to flex the whole spine.

(c) Reverse both movements to return to the starting position.

(d) Gently extend the straight leg, and feel the gluteals contracting (14iii).

Teaching Point

The trunk should remain as vertical as possible, i.e. not swing from the hips to counteract the leg.

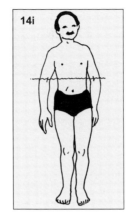
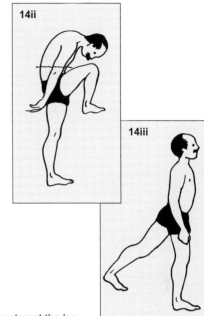

15. ROWING

Why do it?

To increase flexion and extension in the whole spine. To improve balance and to work the upper trunk and arm muscles.

Starting position

Stand with the feet shoulder-width apart in chest-high water.

Movement

(a) Keeping the knees straight at all times, reach as far as possible in front, as though stretching holding some oars (15i). In order not to overbalance, it is necessary to stick the buttock out to the rear.

(b) Perform an imaginary rowing movement by pulling back with the arms and trunk. As the knees are still straight, in order not to overbalance it is necessary to move the centre part of the body forwards, thereby arching the lumbar spine and extending the hips (15ii).

(c) Continue rowing without toppling over!

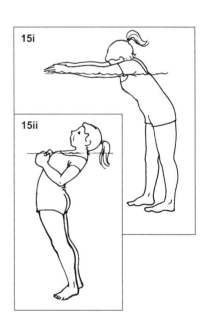

Variation

This exercise works well in pairs. The couple face each other, standing a little way apart. There are then two options; they can both reach forward together to approximate their hands, or they can imagine that they are holding short pieces of rope in each hand, so that as one person pulls backwards, they pull the other person forwards, and vice versa.

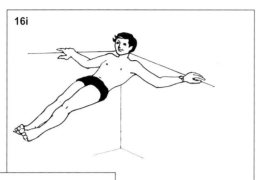

16i

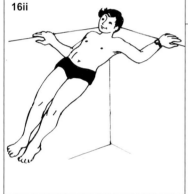

16ii

16iii

16iv

16. THE FIGUREHEAD

Why do it?

It is a really useful exercise as it not only helps spinal flexibility, but also works the back extensor, leg and buttock muscles. The arm muscles also work to stabilize the body. It is pleasant to do, but it **must be used with extreme caution by back sufferers whose pain is aggravated by extension**. It can, though, even relieve a mild ache in some circumstances. In summary it combines active and passive flexion and extension.

Limitation

It can only be done if there is a firm anchor point on which to place the head, and a rail or other place to hold on to. A corner is ideal, but if not available it is sometimes possible to be positioned along the side of a pool.

Starting position

Lie supine, floating on the surface (without buoyancy aids), but assisted by the arms helping to maintain the horizontal position. The head must be wedged against the pool wall, rail or corner (16i).

Movement

(a) Keeping the umbilicus on (or above) the surface of the water as long as possible, extend the spine by pulling downwards leading with both legs. The knees should remain straight. The head acts as a fulcrum and the whole of the spine should arch downwards and backwards from that point, for as long as possible (16ii).

(b) Continue until standing on the feet.

(c) Now change the grip if necessary, and still holding on and keeping the feet in the same place, take the trunk forwards, so as to be in the position of the emblem lady on a Rolls Royce or the Figurehead on the front of a Viking ship. Hold that position, and increase the stretch on the lumbar spine, by thrusting the pelvis forwards (16iii).

(d) Now pull the body back with the hands, and change the grip if necessary. Wedge the head, and tuck the knees up towards the chest (16iv). When the heels are on the surface, then extend both legs, to return to the starting position.

(e) Repeat all the stages, slowly, several times.

Teaching points

In order to prevent straining in the shoulders, the head must be the fulcrum. Sometimes, when repeating the exercise, the downward movement is started before the head is fixed, and this is potentially hazardous.

17. WALL SQUATS

Requirement

A bar to hold on to.

Why do it?

Squats are a great way to increase lumbar flexion and stretch the hamstrings and sciatic nerve. This exercise also feels pleasurably primitive!

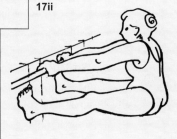

Starting position

Hold onto the bar and place the feet up against the side-wall of the pool, with the feet pointing outwards. Make sure that the knees are always directly over the feet, thereby preventing twisting of the knees.

Movement

(a) Pull on the hands to increase the hip and knee flexion. Try to have the legs in as much outward rotation, flexion and abduction as possible (in a true 'squat'), so that the hands are inside the knees (17i).

(b) Gently push on the feet to try and straighten the knees (17ii). This needs to be done with caution, observing the Pain Principle, as it can aggravate a sciatic lesion. If there is normal flexibility, and no pathology, it is usually possible to push against the wall and lift the buttocks almost out of the water.

Precaution

This exercise should be performed slowly, in the client's own time, without inflicting a rhythm on them.

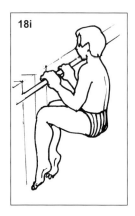
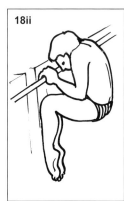

18. WALL KNEELS

Requirement

A bar to hold on to.

Why do it?

To increase spinal flexion.

Starting position

Hold onto the bar. Place one leg against the side of the pool so that the foot is maximally plantar flexed, then bring the other leg up to match (18i).

Movement

(a) Pull gently with the hands so as to try and curl up into a little ball, by sitting on one's heels and trying to get the chin to touch the bar (18ii).

(b) Push away with the hands against the wall, to return to the kneeling position.

19. BARRE TUCKS

This exercise is similar to Squat tucks, but is more localized to the lumbosacral junction. It is particularly appropriate when pregnant.

Why do it?

To flex fully the lumbosacral junction, and increase awareness of the perineum.

Starting position

Hold onto the side, with the hands together. Bring the feet up so that you are squatting on the side of the pool. Try to get the feet flat against the wall (19i).

Movement

Increase the knee flexion and at the same time bend forwards (19ii), as though trying to see whether a baby is being born!

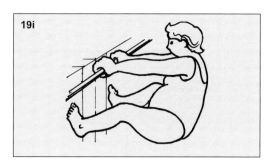

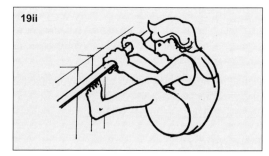

20. HORIZONTAL TUCKS

Why do it?

To increase lumbar flexion.

Starting position

Lie on your back, supported by floats if necessary (20i).

Movement

(a) Keeping your knees and feet together, bring both knees up towards your chest (20ii).

(b) Return to the starting position.

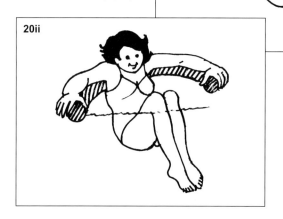

EXERCISES THAT PRIMARILY INVOLVE SIDE FLEXION

21. SIDE BENDS WITH REACHES

Why do it?

To increase rotation and side flexion in the lumbar spine.

Starting position

Stand with the feet wide apart, preferably in waist-high water.

Movement

(a) Reach as far as possible sideways to the right with the right hand, so that the hand pushes away the surface of the water (21i).

(b) Rotate the pelvis towards the right side, as the left arm follows the right arm (21ii).

(c) Reverse the movements to return to the starting position.

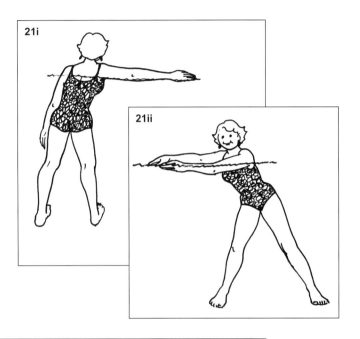

22. WAIST LINE

Why do it?

To gain trunk side-mobility (and it might help the waist-line!).

Starting position

Stand in chest-high water with the legs apart. Place the right hand in the waist, and the left hand on the surface of the water, to the side.

Movement

(a) With the left hand, draw an imaginary line on the surface of the water, stretching over to the right. At the same time, create some counter-pressure by pushing the right hand into the waist – to act as a fulcrum for the movement. Allow the pelvis to be pushed to the left – to maintain balance (22ii). This stretches the waist.

(b) Reverse the movement to return to the starting position. Repeat to the same side several times, before reversing directions.

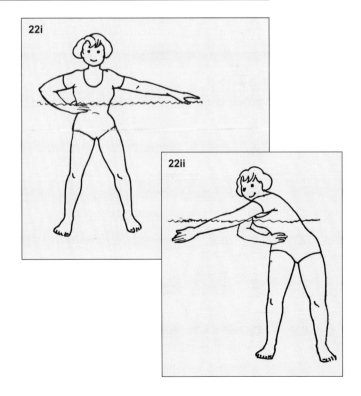

23. HORIZONTAL SIDE BENDS

Why do it? To increase side flexion.

Starting position

Lie supine, preferably in a corner. If no corner is available, then hold on to the sides with your hands as wide apart as possible, and float on your back.

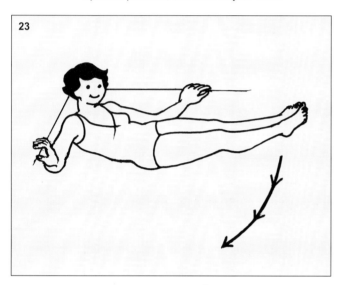

23

Movement

(a) In the corner, trying to keep your trunk parallel to the surface, and your belly-button just above the surface of the water, and more or less stationary all the time, bend from the waist to swing your lower body in one piece to one side, so that you are trying to make your ankle bones touch the wall. Keep your feet together all the time.

(b) If no corner is available, then swing your lower body to an angle of 45 degrees from the mid-line, so that your torso makes a kind of horizontal pendulum, but only below the waist.

(c) If the pool is deep enough, this exercise can also be done vertically, in imitation of a pendular movement. In which case it should be called vertical side bends!

24. FACET PUSHES

Why do it?

This exercise is designed to mobilize the facet or epiphyseal joints at the sides of the lumbar vertebrae which are particularly prone to degenerative changes.

Starting position

Stand with the feet shoulder-width apart, and the right hand placed on the right upper thigh or buttock, in chest-high water.

Movement

(a) Run the right hand down the back of the right leg, by tipping backwards from the waist (24ii).

(b) Then stand up.

(c) Reach diagonally forwards and outwards with the left hand, along the surface of the water (24iii).

(d) Return to the starting position.

(e) Repeat the whole pattern several times to one side before changing directions.

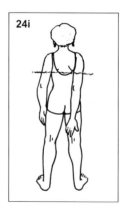

24i

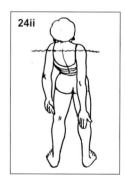

24ii

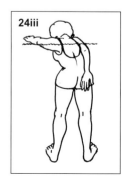

24iii

C ABDOMINALS EXERCISES

These exercises are all aimed at improving muscle function. It is important to stress that the *tummy should be well pulled in at all times*, in order to work the transversis abdominis, arguably the most important of the abdominal muscles.

Almost all of these exercises are performed lying in the supine position, supported by holding on to the side, or with the help of floats. They are all designed to work the abdominal muscles.

EXERCISES WHICH PRIMARILY WORK RECTUS ABDOMINIS

These are arranged in order of difficulty.

25. CYCLING

Starting position Lie on your back, trying to be as flat as possible, preferably with the head supported.

Movement

Perform a cycling motion with the legs, keeping them mostly underneath the water. Imagine the pedals are a little longer than usual, so that the cycling motion can be a bit larger.

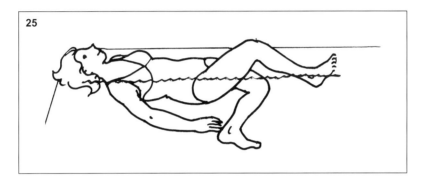

26. TOE-OUT CURLS

Starting position Lie on your back with both legs stretched out straight, and the feet pulled at the ankle joints.

Movement

(a) Keeping the toes out of the water at all times, pull both knees up towards you, as though you are getting into a crunch position. Imagine that your toes will melt if they get wet!

(b) Slowly return to the starting position, still keeping your toes dry.

Progression

Do the exercise more slowly!

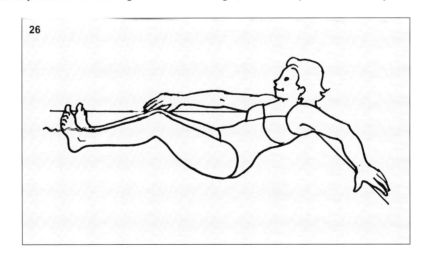

27. ALTERNATE TOE-OUT CURLS

Starting position

Lie on your back with one leg stretched out straight, and the other pulled up as far as possible.

Movement

Whilst keeping your toes out of the water at all times, bend one leg while the other one is straightening, alternating legs.

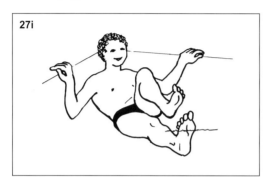

28. PRONE SCISSORS

Starting position

Lie on your tummy, either supported on floats, or held up in the horizontal position by having one hand pushing you up and away from the wall, whilst the other hand holds on to the side.

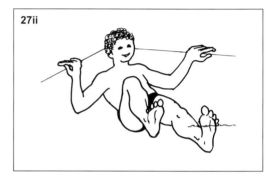

Movement

Keeping your knees straight at all times, perform a scissoring movement with your legs. Open the scissors as wide as possible, and move your legs quickly from the top to the bottom position.

29. SIT SCISSORS

Starting position

Hold yourself onto the side-wall of the pool, so that your bottom is against the wall, but your legs are stretched out in front of you, with the knees straight (29i).

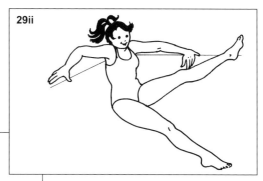

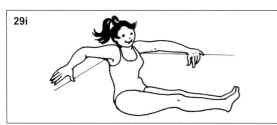

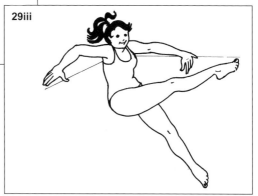

Movement

(a) Lift up one straight leg, whilst lowering the other one, so as to part the legs in a vertical plane.

(b) Keep scissoring and feel your tummy working.

30. PANCAKE TUCKS

Requirement

Buoyancy aids, e.g. floats, woggles or empty bottles to assist with flotation.

Why do it?

To improve range of motion by doing a full range movement, in a pleasing way.

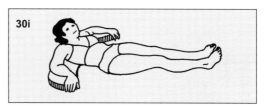

Starting position

With the help of the buoyancy aids, float on your back, with your feet together (30i).

Movement

(a) Pull both knees as far up to the chest as possible (as you do this your bottom will sink down a little) (30ii).

(b) Roll forwards so that you are lying prone. Push the legs out straight behind you (30iv).

(c) Tuck the knees in and tip backwards to return to the starting position. You are tossing the pancake.

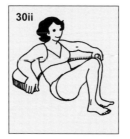

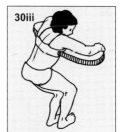

Variation

If the pool is deep enough, you can add an extra tuck in and push down with an intervening vertical thrust.

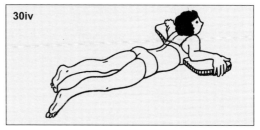

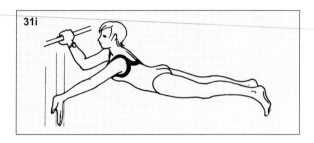

31. PRONE BODY TUCKS

Starting position

Lie on your tummy, holding on with one hand on the rail or the outside (in a deck level pool), and the other hand positioned so that the palm is against the wall and the heel of the hand is up, to help you maintain the horizontal prone position (31i).

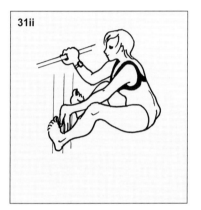

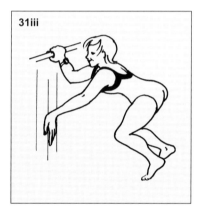

Movement

(a) Leading with the knees, bring both legs up and flex at the hips so that you are squatting against the side (31ii).

(b) Extend your spine and take your hips back, following with your legs (31iii) to return to the starting position.

32. PRONE KNEE CURLS

Starting position

As for the previous exercise.

Movement

Almost the same as the previous exercise, but this time end up kneeling against the side wall, instead of squatting.

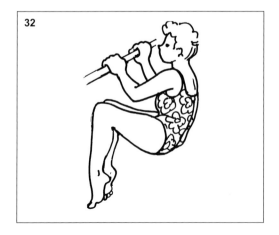

33. PIKE LIFT (with floats)

Starting position

This is the one time that you can mimic the Olympic gymnasts! Put a strong float under each hand, and push down on them. Lift up both straight legs to be in the Pike position.

Movement

(a) Keeping the knees straight and together, lift both legs up so that the feet come out of the water.

(b) To return to the starting position, you will need to flex the knees and hips, and push both legs straight down underneath you.

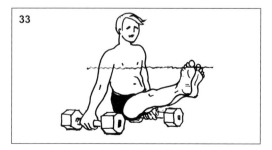

EXERCISES WHICH WORK THE ABDOMINAL OBLIQUE MUSCLES

The tummy **must** be pulled in tightly.

34. HELICOPTERS

Requirement Floats under the arms.

Starting position

Hang from floats, with the knees bent.

Movement

(a) Turn over towards one side and make a cycle movement with both legs also tipped to the side. Keep the trunk more or less vertical. You should find that you turn around on your own axis.

(b) Reverse direction by tipping towards the other side.

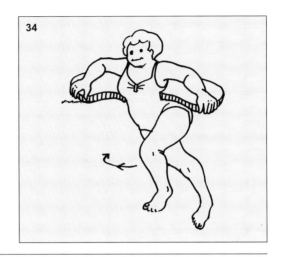

35. TWISTS

Starting position

Lie on your back, supported by floats, or by holding on to the sides, or a corner. Bend up both knees, so that they are out of the water. Keep the knees and feet touching each other.

Movement

Tip both knees over to one side, then over to the other side. Try to end up with the pelvis rotated at right angles to the chest. This exercise can also be done lying supine with the arms extended, holding floats to maintain the position. One leg can be lifted right out of the water, whilst the other descends. The entire trunk should remain horizontal and not 'dip'.

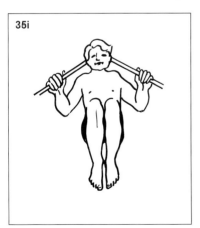
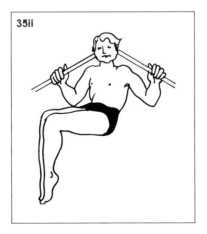
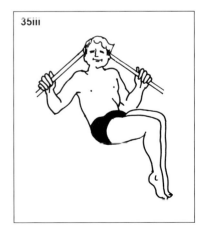

36. RESISTED SPOON CORKSCREW

Starting position

Stand in chest-high water with the feet apart, and the knees a little bent. Lift your hands up to the surface, and form them into spoon-shapes (36i).

Movement

(a) Turn your upper body round as if trying to look behind you. As you move, use you hands as 'spoons' to make a little wall of water as you turn – both 'spoons' facing towards the direction of the movement.

(b) Turn round as far as you can, then reverse the direction of the movement, and of the spoons.

(c) Keep your knees facing forwards, fixing the hips, so that it is the trunk that moves, so working the abdominals.

(d) Repeat from side to side, with as large a movement as possible. You should be able to see the same spot in the wall behind you, from either direction!

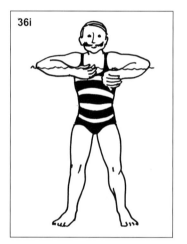 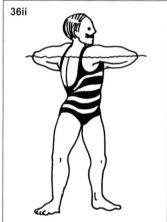 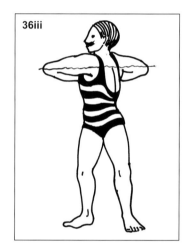

37. RESISTED PADDLE CORKSCREW

Starting position:

Stand in chest-high water, with your knees a little bent, the trunk vertical and both hands on hips.

Movement

Rotate from the waist, as in previous exercise, but this time feel the additional drag caused by the elbows, which are acting somewhat like paddle-boat wheels.

Teaching Point

Try not to move the shoulder joints. The arms and trunk should move in one piece.

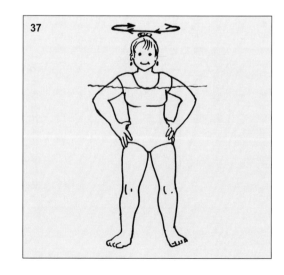

38. U-TUCKS

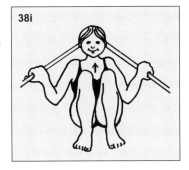

38i

Starting position

This exercise is a progression of Exercise 35 (The Twists). The starting position is the same.

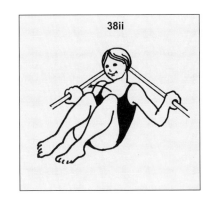

38ii

Movement

This time, instead of merely flipping the legs over from side to side, do it in a slower, more controlled way and make a small reverse U-shape with your knees, by tucking them up towards your chin, in a semi-lunar scoop.

39. PARTS AND CROSSOVERS

Starting position

Lie floating on your back with the legs stretched out straight. You may need some help from floats, or from holding on to the corner.

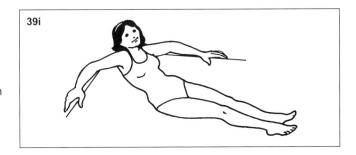

39i

Movement

(a) Open your legs as wide apart as possible.
(b) Bring them together, and twist from the waist bringing your left hip out of the water.
     Keep moving your legs in the same direction, so that your left leg crosses over your right leg.
     Try to get them as wide apart when crossed over, as they were when just parted.
(c) Reverse direction so as to part them again as widely as possibly.
(d) Cross over again, but this time going the other way, with the right leg leading and the right hip lifting.

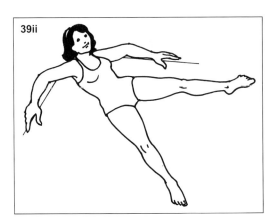

39ii

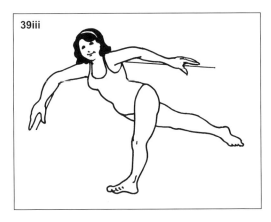

39iii

40. V-SHAPES

This is a very hard exercise that works the abdominals, as well as everything else!

Starting position

Lie floating on your back, either in the corner of a pool with your head wedged, or with a woggle under the small of your back for support. Bend both knees up onto your chest (40i).

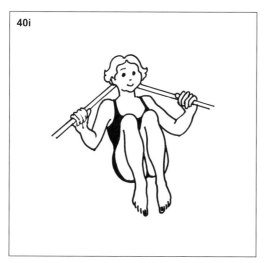

40i

Movement

(a) Twist your spine so that both legs flip over to the left (40ii).

(b) Straighten both knees, so that your entire body is aligned to the wall of the pool (40iii).

(c) Reverse the movement, so as to bring both knees up from the left side (40iv).

(d) When you get up as far as possible, flip the whole lower body over to the right side.

(e) Stretch both knees and your body out against the right pool wall (40v).

(f) Continue so that your lower body describes a V-shape going through an angle of 45 degrees to either side of the midline.

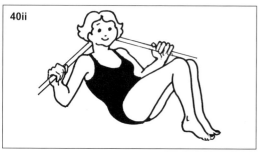

40ii

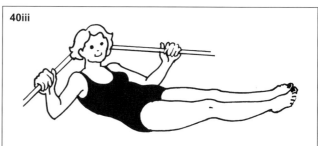

40iii

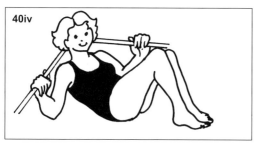

40iv

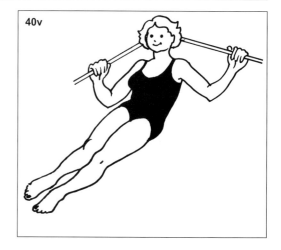

40v

Teaching point

If you do this exercise on floats, instead of holding on to the side, you will find that the leg movement is diminished, but the upper body moves in the opposite direction instead.

D UPPER QUADRANT

Shoulder, Girdle and Arm Exercises

For mobility, and as warm-up exercises.

41. SHOULDER SHRUGS

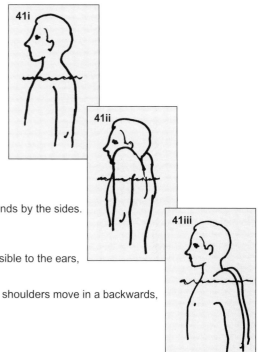

Why do it?

- To mobilize the joints in the shoulder girdle and upper spine.
- To reduce tension in the trapezius muscle.
- To improve postural awareness.

Starting position

Stand in shoulder-high water, with the feet just a little apart, and the hands by the sides.

Movements

(a) Shrug both shoulders up so as to get the shoulders as near as possible to the ears, then lower them so as to make the neck as long as possible.

(b) Round both shoulders, then pull them back, so that the point of the shoulders move in a backwards, forwards direction. Feel the movement between the shoulder blades.

Teaching points

Make sure that the neck is long, and the chin is not poking forwards (41iii).

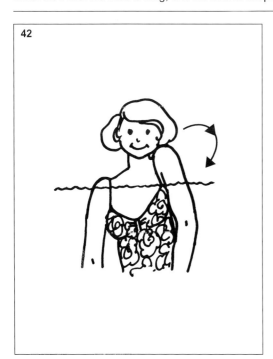

42. BACKWARDS AND FORWARDS SHOULDER CIRCLES

Starting position

Stand with the legs apart in water that is just on the point of the shoulders. If the water is not deep enough, then bend the knees.

Movement

(a) Lift one shoulder out of the water and roll it backwards to make a circle. The arm should remain relaxed so that it is carried round by the point of the shoulder.

(b) Reverse the direction of the circle to make it forwards.

Variations

The shoulders can circle separately or together. If together, they can go in the same direction, or in opposite directions.

43. HUGGING

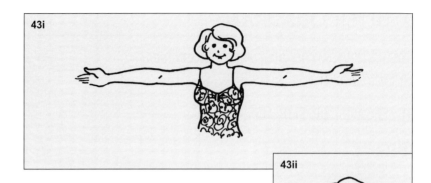

Starting position

Position yourself so that the water is just below shoulder level. Stretch both arms out to the side, so that they are floating on the surface with the palms facing forwards.

Movement

(a) Keeping your elbows nearly straight, bring both hands together as though you were going to clap.

(b) Allow the hands to cross over and keep moving in the same direction, so that you end up hugging yourself.

(c) Reverse the direction to return to the starting position.

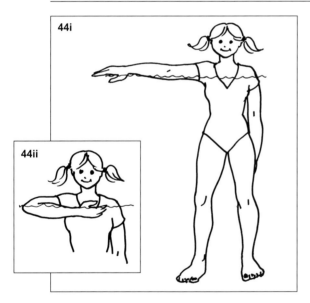

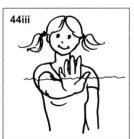

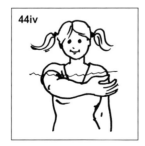

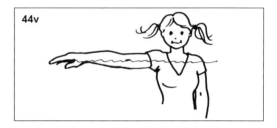

44. OUT AND ACROSS

Starting position

Stand with the feet apart, for stability, in shoulder-high water. Stretch the right arm, palm down, out to the side as far as possible (44i).

Movement

(a) Flex the right arm in towards the centre of the chest (44ii), then push it away with the heel of the hand, making a little wall of water, and aiming diagonally across and in front of you, directly in line with the left shoulder (44iii).

(b) Reverse the motion, by turning over your hand and using your palm to pull water in to your chest (44iv).

(c) Finally, push out to return to the starting position.

(d) Reverse arms either alternately, or after a 'set'.

45. CUTTING A DIAMOND

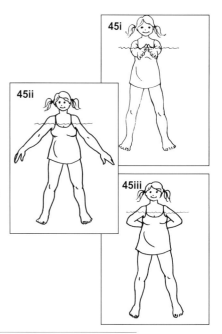

Why do it? To mobilize and stabilize the shoulder region.

Starting position

Stand with the feet apart in shoulder-high water, with both hands stretched out in front, index fingers touching so as to make a roof shape, with the thumbs up as the chimneys (45i).

Movement

(a) Keeping the arms and fingers straight, draw both arms downwards and outwards (making the top half of a diamond shape) and stopping when the arms make an angle of 45 degrees to the body – the diamond position (45ii).

(b) Holding the upper arms in exactly the same position, flex the elbows so that the back of the hands gets as close as possible to waist level.

(c) Still holding the upper arms in the same position, straighten the elbows out again, to return the diamond position.

(d) Return to starting position, by cutting a reverse diamond pattern through the water.

46. ARM WALKING

This exercise involves active and passive stretching.

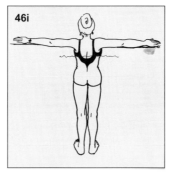

Starting position

Stand facing the side of the pool and hold on with both hands, arms as wide apart as possible (46i).

Movement

(a) The aim of this exercise is to move around the edge of the pool, turning as you do so, but keeping alternate hands stationary as an anchor around which you pivot.

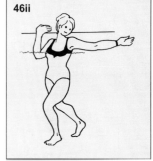

(b) When moving to the right around the pool, release the left hand and swing it behind you, followed by the rest of your body, so that your body is turning in an anticlockwise direction (46ii).

(c) Keep going until the left hand can grab the side, as far away from the right hand as is comfortable, so you are facing away from the edge (46iii).

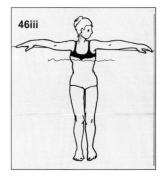

(d) Now release your right hand and continue turning the body in the same anticlockwise direction until that hand can catch hold of the side. You are now back in the starting position, but further to the right around the pool side. You obviously have to stop if the water gets too deep for safety. If so, then reverse the direction of movement so that you are moving to the left and performing clockwise circles.

Variations The further apart your hands, the more the stretch on the arms and shoulders.

• The quicker the movement is done, the harder you work your muscles.
• The maximum stretch to the shoulder is achieved by having the arms as high as possible. To achieve this either move to deeper water or bend your knees.

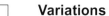

47. ELBOW CIRCLES

Starting position

Stand, with the feet a little way apart, and place both hands so that they are just touching the point of the corresponding shoulders.

Movement

Circle both elbows, making as large a movement as possible.

Variations

- Circle clockwise and anticlockwise.
- Circle so that the arms are working in the same direction and in opposing directions.

48. HAND FIGURE-OF-EIGHT

This is primarily a mobility exercise for the radio-ulnar and wrist joints, but also involves some shoulder rotation.

Starting position

Stand with the elbows pushed into the waist and the joints at 90 degrees. The right palm should be facing upwards, and the left one downwards. Keep the feet apart for stability (48i).

Movement

(a) Keeping the elbows in contact with the waist at all times, take both hands to the right (externally rotating the right shoulder and internally rotating the left).

(b) Keeping the wrist joint in neutral, perform a figure-of-eight movement with both forearms and hands (48ii).

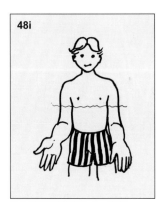

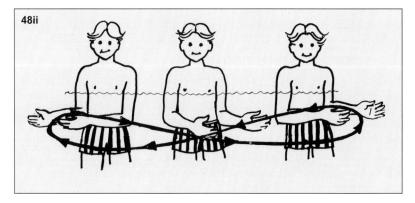

49. TENNIS SWINGS

Starting position

Stand with the feet apart.

Movement

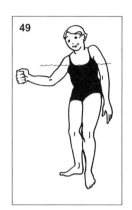

(a) Move the arm as though making an imaginary forehand or backhand tennis stroke.

(b) Make it harder by keeping the wrist fixed in neutral, and holding the fingers together.

(c) Make it even harder by swinging with a plastic bat (with plastic stringing).

(d) Repeat with the non-dominant arm.

50. GOLF SWINGS

Starting position

The golfers will know how to stand.

Movement

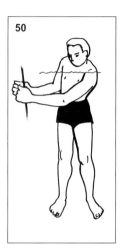

A pretend golf drive, holding an imaginary club. Do not forget the follow through. Try it to the other side, as though left-handed.

The Arm and Shoulder Girdle

The following exercises are primarily for muscular training.

51. SEA-HORSING

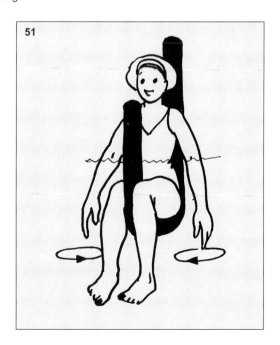

Requirement

A woggle, or other buoyancy device that will permit the sitting position without impeding movement.

Starting position

Place the woggle between the legs, with slightly more of it behind you, so that the front end does not hit you on the chin. Sit on it, bringing your legs up. Keep your trunk vertical as though riding a monocycle.

Movement

Move yourself around the pool by paddling only with your arms. It is not as easy as it sounds, as it requires excellent trunk control not to overbalance and fairly hard arm exertion in order to move quickly.

52. WALL PRESS-UPS

Requirement

Something to hold on to.

Muscles working

Triceps, biceps.

Starting position

Stand facing the wall, holding on to a bar, or the edge of the pool, with the feet together.

Movement

(a) Keeping your trunk and legs in a straight line, pull your body forward with your hands, so that you flex both elbows, until your chin touches the bar.

(b) Then push away from the bar with both hands, back to the starting position. This is a very easy version of a press-up. It should be done quickly, to take advantage of the water resistance.

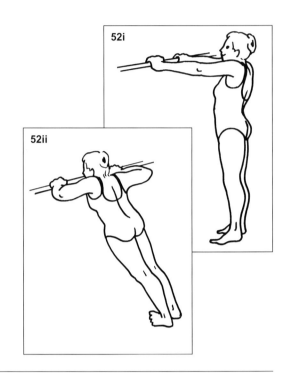

53. PECTORAL ARMS

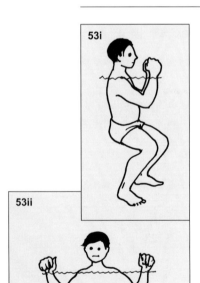

Muscles working

• Going forward: pectorals and anterior deltoid.

• Going backwards: rhomboids and lower trapezius and latissimus dorsi.

Starting position

Bend your knees, so that the water is just below the chin. The elbows must be held so that the forearms are vertical throughout. Have both elbows, forearms and fists touch each other centrally (53i).

Movement

(a) Using the trunk muscles to stabilize the spine, take both elbows out to the side as far as possible, so that you can feel a tightening between the shoulder blades (53ii). In order to get as much of the forearm as possible in the water and increase the resistance, allow the elbows to drop a little.

(b) When as far out as possible, reverse the movement, so that the forearms touch each other.

Variations

Increase the speed and/or put an unstreamlined object around the arm below the elbow to increase water resistance.

54. ARM SWINGING

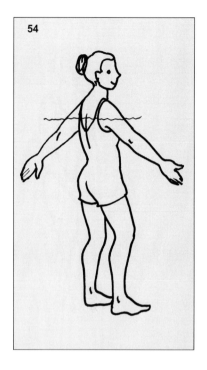

Muscles working

Biceps and triceps, anterior and posterior fibres of deltoid, and others.

Starting position

Stand with the feet just a little apart with one in front of the other.

Movement

(a) Keeping the elbows straight, and the hands and fingers in a straight line (thumbs forward) swing one arm forwards at the same time as you swing the other arm backwards.

(b) Reverse directions. This is an imitation of the arm movements when marching, but the feet keep still. It is much harder work to stand still than to move the legs, especially if the arms move quickly.

Progression

1. Turn the hands round so as to get additional resistance.

2. Move the arms more quickly.

3. Wear glove flippers.

55. BICEPS–TRICEPS CURLS

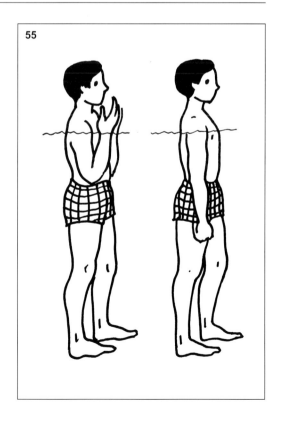

Starting position

Stand with the elbows pushed into the waist and the joints at 90 degrees. Both palms should be facing upwards. Keep the feet apart for stability.

Movement

(a) Keeping the elbows pressed into the waist, the wrist joint in a neutral position and the fingers together and aligned with the forearm, flex both elbows so that the palms approximate to the shoulders. This works the biceps.

(b) Extend to straighten the elbow joints, but still keeping the wrist and hand in a straight line. This works the triceps.

Variations

Have one elbow flexing as the other one is extending.

Progression

Make it harder by wearing gloves or flippers. The muscle work will change if you hold buoyant objects.

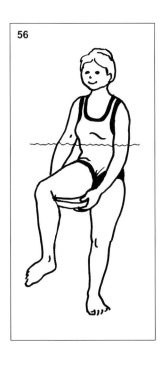

56. FLOAT OR FRISBEE CIRCLES

Muscles working

Latissimus dorsi (if floats) and most other muscles of the arms and upper trunk, –depending on exactly how the exercise is done and whether the float is buoyant or a frisbee-type object.

Starting position

Stand with the feet together. Lift up one leg so that the thigh is horizontal and the lower leg is dangling down.

Movement

(a) Pass the frisbee or float around the thigh. Angle it so that it is hard to push through the water.

(b) Pass it several times round one thigh, balancing on one leg as you are doing this.

(c) Repeat with the other leg.

(d) Pass them round alternate thighs, so that the object makes a figure-of-eight as it goes around your legs.

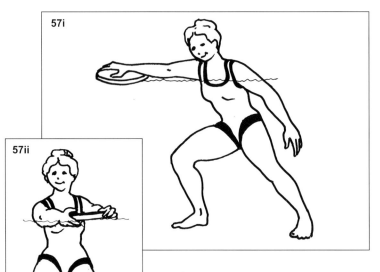

57. FRISBEE PASSES

Muscles working

Most of the arm and shoulder girdle muscles, especially the pectorals.

Starting position

Stand with the feet wide apart. Hold an object, like a plastic plate or a frisbee in the right hand, bend the right knee, and stretch out as far as you can to the right. The left hand will come up to assist in balance (57i).

Movement

(a) Pull the float towards you until it is in front of you, then transfer it to your left hand and continue moving it to the left (57ii).

(b) You should feel the movement happening from the feet, and find that the knees are flexing and extending, in order to get the maximum stretch without over-balancing.

(c) The faster you move, the harder the work!

58. SIDE CIRCLES

Muscles working

All of them.

Starting position

Stand with the feet wide apart in chest- to shoulder-depth water.

Movement

(a) Imagine your arm is a pen, and your index finger is the nib. Draw enormous circles to the sides, the front and in as many other different planes as possible.

(b) You are allowed to bring your arm out of the water so as to reach above your head.

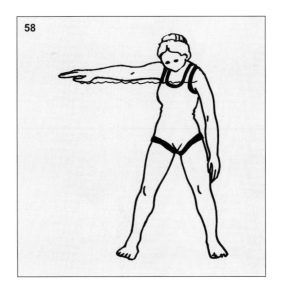

59. BICEPS PUMP

Muscle working

Biceps – concentrically coming down (59i) and eccentrically when going up (59ii).

Starting position

Stand with the legs apart in shoulder-high water with one arm stretched out on the surface to the side, with the back of your hand uppermost. Hold a buoyant object such as an empty fabric conditioner bottle with the lid on, or a knotted woggle.

Movement

(a) Without moving the upper arm, slowly bend your elbow so that you bring the 'float' down towards your waist.

(b) Reverse the movement, to allow the float to move up in a slow, controlled way.

Progression

Take the arms further behind you, so that the elbows are flexing more in a forward–backwards plane.

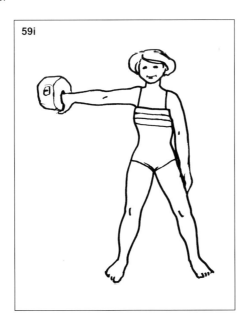

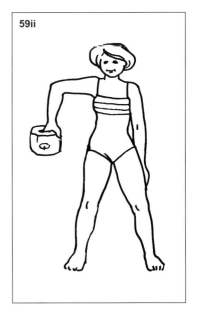

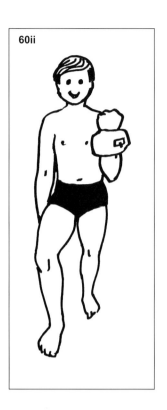

60. TRICEPS PUMP

Muscles working

Triceps – eccentrically coming up and concentrically when going down.

Starting position

Stand with the feet apart, one foot behind the other. Bend the right knee. Place the back of your right hand on your thigh, with your elbow fixed into your waist. Hold a buoyant object in the left hand or wear blown-up armbands around the wrist.

Movement

(a) Slowly flex the left elbow, but keep the elbow in contact with the waist.

(b) When the elbow is fully bent, then slowly push it down to straighten the arm.

(c) This may be possible working both arms at the same time, but one needs to come up as the other one goes down, and it may depend on the buoyancy of the person and the object.

61. TRICEPS LIFT

Muscles working

Triceps, trapezius and rhomboids.

Starting position

This depends on the design of the pool. If the distance between the water level and the surrounding surface is not too great, then hold on to the top of the pool (or a bar if there is one). Preferably have your back to the wall, so that your elbows are bent behind you (61i). Alternatively, face the wall.

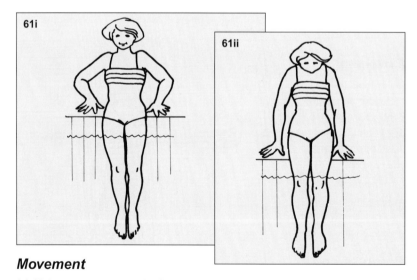

Movement

(a) Using your arms, slowly lift your body out of the water.

(b) Slowly lower your body down, keeping control.

(c) Do not jump up, but do this as a controlled lift up using only the arms.

(d) Repeat, trying to tire out the muscle.

62. PECTORAL AND LOW TRAP SQUEEZES

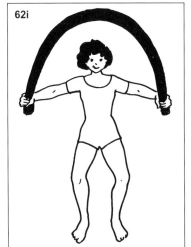

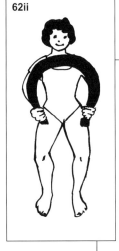

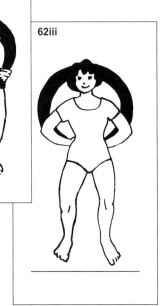

Requirement

A woggle.

Starting position

Stand with the feet apart for stability, and the knees slightly bent, in chest-high water. Hold the ends of the woggle as illustrated (62i).

Movement

(a) Push both ends together (62ii) so that they touch to the front of you, hold for the count of 5 (keeping the tummy pulled in), then slowly release.

(b) Repeat, but this time, try and get the ends to touch behind you, at buttock level (62iii).

E LOWER QUADRANT

Pelvis and Legs – for Mobility

THE CHANGES (p. 140)

This exercise is particularly effective for the lower limbs as it facilitates a normal walking pattern.

63. ONE LEG MARCHING

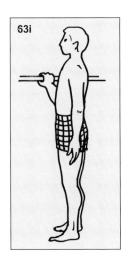

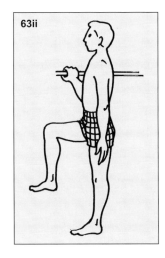

Starting position

Stand erect, with the feet together, like a Guardsman on sentry duty. Remember to pull in the tummy and maintain perfect body alignment. Hold on with one hand.

Movement

(a) Pick up one leg, so that the hip and knee come to a right angle.

(b) Push the leg back down to its starting position.

(c) Repeat with the other leg, so you are marching on the spot.

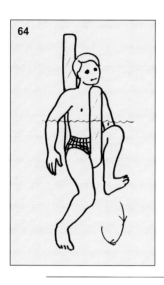

64. WOGGLE CYCLING

Requirement

A woggle, or other buoyancy device that will permit the sitting position without impeding movement.

Starting position

Place the woggle between the legs, with slightly more of it behind you, so that the front end does not hit you on the chin. Sit on it, bringing your legs up. Keep your trunk vertical as though riding a monocycle.

Movement

(a) Move yourself around the pool by cycling only with your legs and feet.

(b) Try going round in circles, or in different directions, always without losing balance and tipping over.

65. STEAM ENGINE CIRCLES

Why do it?

This is a particularly good exercise, as it works hips and knees through a full range of flexion and extension.

Explanation

This exercise is so called, because the legs perform a kind of elliptical, egg-shaped 'circle', that is reminiscent of the movement that happens with the pistons of a steam train.

Starting position

Hold on to the side with your left hand. Bring the straight right leg up in front of you.,

Movement

(a) Pull the straight right leg backwards, until the leg is behind you.

(b) Flex the right knee, as though trying to kick your own right buttock.

(c) Keeping the knee flexed, take the bent knee forwards, until it is tucked up in front of you.

(d) Keep the thigh still and kick out the lower leg to complete the circle and return to the start.

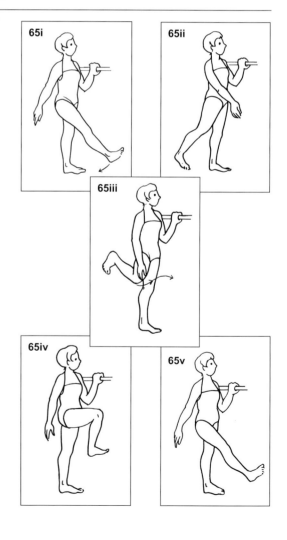

66. WEIGHT TRANSFER WITH REACHES

Why do it?

This is a functional exercise, that helps with balance, as well as mobilizing the hips and knees.

Starting position

Stand with the feet at least shoulder-width apart, and the hands on the surface.

Movement

(a) Lean on the right foot, and as you transfer the weight onto it, bend the right knee and reach with your hands as far as possible out to the right (66i).

(b) Straighten the left leg to help you maintain your balance.

(c) If you are comfortable doing that, allow the left leg to lift up and stretch out when you are in the extreme position (66ii).

(d) Return to the starting position, and repeat to the opposite side.

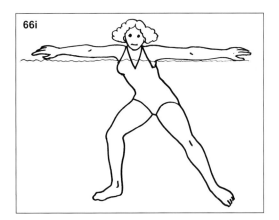

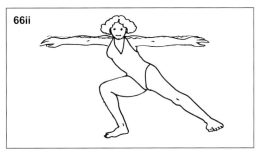

67. STEP LUNGES

Requirement

A step. This can be either a step built into the structure of the pool, at a depth of up to one metre, or it could be an aquastep (i.e. a step used for an aquatic step class)

Why do it?

It increases the range of movement in the ankle and knee joints. It is a functional exercise – a preliminary to going up and down stairs.

Starting position

Stand with the feet apart, one in front of the other – with one leg one or two levels above the other leg, on a step. Keep both feet flat all the time.

Movement

(a) Lean on the left leg, so as to lunge forward and increase the flexion.

(b) Return to the standing position.

(c) Lean on the back leg, but keep the front foot flat, so that the ankle joint is as straight as possible.

(d) Make it more interesting by pretending to do a sword thrust with the arm, as you lunge forwards.

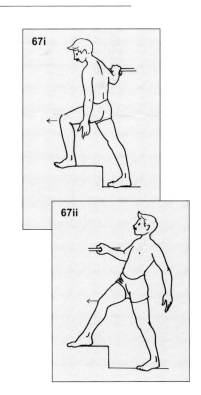

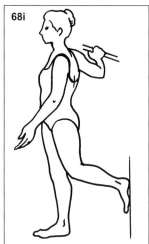

68. WALL PUSHES

Why do it?

This exercise is a closed chain movement for the knee, which mobilizes the knee joint. Because it is unusual to be pushing off from the back, there are less inhibitions which therefore assists mobilization of a stiff knee.

Starting position

Stand facing away from the wall, but hold on with the right hand. Place the left foot against the wall, so that the foot is vertical. Place the toes at the level of the other ankle.

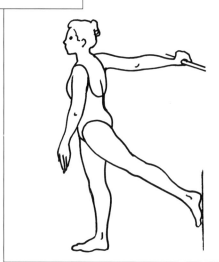

Movement

Push away from the wall with the left foot, but do not push too hard, as you need to restrain yourself from pushing away with the right hand When the right arm is straight, use the hand to pull yourself back to the starting position. Be careful not to twist the knee.

69. CAN CAN

Precaution

The knee is thought of as a hinge joint, but when flexed, there is a certain amount of rotation. This must not be done with a knee which locks, or in the presence of any pain.

Why do it?

To increase range of movement in the knee joint. To help re-train balance (if not holding on!).

Starting position

Stand on one leg, holding on only if necessary, lift up one leg, and bend the knee to a right angle.

Movement

(a) Circle the lower part of the leg (as if doing the can-can). The rotation should take place below the knee and in the thigh.

(b) Reverse direction. Change legs.

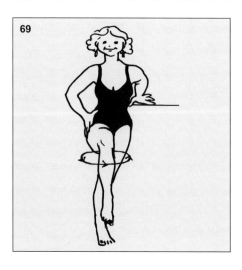

FOR IMPROVING MUSCLE FUNCTION

As many of the exercises are complicated and involve functional movements, rather than single joint movements, they are subdivided according to the type of movement:

- HIP AND/OR KNEE: FLEXION AND EXTENSION
- HIP AND/OR KNEE: ABDUCTION AND ADDUCTION
- ROTATION

HIP AND/OR KNEE: FLEXION AND EXTENSION

70. STRAIGHT LEG SWINGING

Why do it?

- Do it slowly and gently to loosen up the hips and lower back.
- Do it quicker to strengthen the muscles in the back, buttock and the thighs.
- Do it very slowly, without holding on, to improve balance.

Starting position

Hold on to the side with one hand, with the body facing at right angles to the wall. Stand straight on the leg nearer the wall.

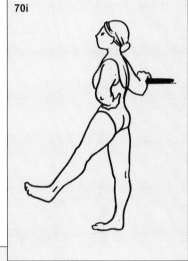

70i

Movement

(a) Brace all the muscles in the other leg, and keeping the knee absolutely straight, swing the stiff leg forwards. Remember, only the leg should move. The head and hips should keep perfectly still.

(b) Now carry the straight leg backwards, so that it is behind you.

Progression

1.   Do a small scale but fast movement, keeping the knee absolutely straight, to strengthen the quadriceps and hip flexors and extensors.

2.   Angle the movement so that the leg moves in either of the two diagonals (forwards and in front of you to backwards and out, or forwards and out to backwards and behind you).

3.   Have the arm on the same side as the leg that is moving also move backwards and forwards, but in the opposite direction (i.e. when the arm is moving forwards, the leg is moving backwards).

4.   Angle the hand so as get maximum water resistance, keeping the fingers together.

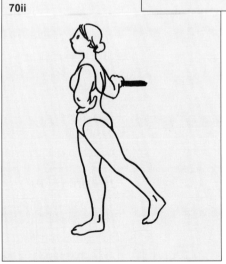

70ii

71. SWIM KICKS

Requirement

For option 1, a float is necessary to support the upper body and stop the arms from moving.

Why do it? To strengthen all the leg muscles and to re-train for swimming.

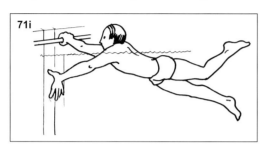

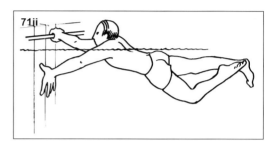

Starting position

Option 1. Lie on your front, holding on to a float, to support the upper body. Keep the body in a straight line.

Option 2. Lie on your front, and hold yourself up by holding on to the side with one hand, while the other hand is placed below you against the wall, and is helping to hold you in the horizontal position.

Movement

(a) Kick with both legs, primarily from the hips, as though doing a 'crawl' leg pattern. The knees should be more or less straight.

(b) If doing option 1, then you can move around the pool. If option 2, this is a stationary manoeuvre.

(c) If this is done wearing flippers, it is likely to make the stationary version harder, but the moving version easier.

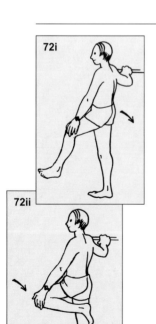

72. EIGHT O'CLOCK KNEE BENDS

Why do it?

To work the major thigh muscles – the quadriceps and the hamstrings.

Starting position

Steady yourself by holding on, unless your balance is excellent! Lift up your left leg and put your hand on your knee. If the hip were the centre of a clock, then the thigh would be at the same angle as the clock would at 8 o'clock (72i).

Movement

Keeping the knee in exactly the same spot, (i.e. without moving your hand), bend and straighten the lower leg and foot (72ii).

Progression

1. Keep the foot pulled up at the ankle joint, so that the foot is rigid. This is the easy version.

2. Let the foot 'flop', i.e. keep the whole foot absolutely relaxed, so that it drags through the water. This is much harder work.

3. Wear a flipper.

73. SUPER-GLUE EXERCISE

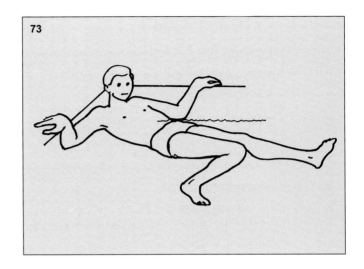

Why do it?

To strengthen and stretch the quadriceps muscle, and to strengthen the hamstrings and the abdominals.

Starting Position

Get into the lying position, so that you are floating on the surface, holding on with your hands. The abdomen should be just below the surface of the water, throughout this exercise. Both knees must remain touching each other, as though glued with superglue, and should stay just below the surface of the water.

Movement

(a) Bend one knee so that foot is brought underneath you, as though trying to kick your own bottom. The exercise is to move the two legs at the same time but in opposite directions, so that one bends as the other straightens.

(b) Remember, the knees themselves should not move, only the leg below the joints. If you do this exercise correctly, then you will feel the pull in the muscle on the front of the thigh.

Variations

For added effect, move quickly and forcefully, letting the foot 'flop' in the water, to give an additional 'drag' factor.

---

74. SUPINE SCISSORS

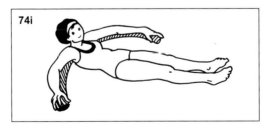

Why do it?

To strengthen the hip and knee flexors and extensors.

Starting position

Lie supine with the legs outstretched.

Movement

(a) Keeping the knee straight at all times, lift one leg up (out of the water).

(b) At the same time, take the other leg down, also keeping it straight.

(c) Alternate the leg action as though scissoring with the legs.

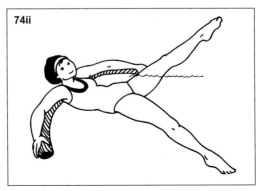

75. FLOOR SQUATS

Why do it?

To strengthen and improve function of the quadriceps and the gluteals.

Starting position

In waist-high water, hold onto the side and stand with the feet a little way apart.

Movement

(a) Go up onto tip-toes (75i).

(b) Bend both knees, letting them move forward as they bend, and keeping the heels raised (75ii).

(c) Stand up, and as you stand feel that you are straightening the knee and putting the heels down.

(d) Repeat the above stages.

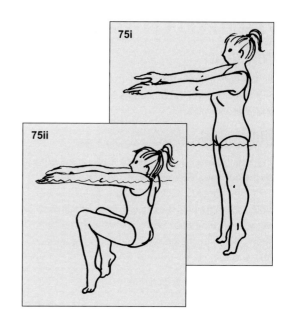

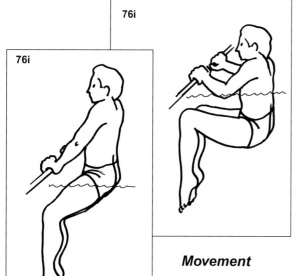

76. WALL KNEEL RISES

Requirement

A bar to hold on to.

Why do it?

To increase work the quadriceps and to increase knee flexion.

Starting position

Hold onto the bar. Place one leg against the side of the pool so that the upper surface of the foot is against the wall, then bring the other leg up to match. Try and get the knees to a right angle or less (76i).

Movement

(a) Push against the wall with your lower legs, so that you lift your head straight up in the air (76ii).

(b) Allow your bottom to lower down as though trying to sit on your heels.

77. STEP-UPS

Why do it?

This is a functional exercise, which should strengthen the quadriceps. Some people who find normal stairs difficult or painful, may be helped by going through the motions in water, where there is less effort, and no pain. In this case, the deeper the water, the easier the exercise is to do.

Starting position

Stand with the right foot up on a step, and the left foot on the step below. The upper foot should always have the heel down (77i).

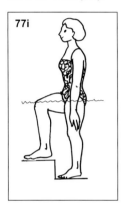
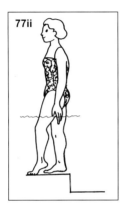

Movement

(a) Step up onto your right leg, making sure to straighten the knee.

(b) Bring up the left foot, and 'tap' the step, so that now both feet are on the upper step (77ii).

(c) Put the left foot down, then take the right foot down and 'tap' the bottom step.

(d) You are ready to lift up the right foot, and keep going.

(e) After 24 step-ups, or so, reverse the feet so that the left goes up first.

78. LUNGES (FENCING PRACTICE)

Why do it? This is an excellent exercise for all-round coordination, balance, and for improving knee function.

Starting position

Stand with your feet almost together, holding an imaginary sword in your right hand.

Movement

(a) Lunge forward so that you land on your right foot, bending the right knee and keeping your back in a straight line (as illustrated). It is important that the knee is placed at the same angle as the foot, to prevent twisting the knee joint. Ideally, foot and knee should be in line with the lunge (78ii).

(b) At the same time make an imaginary forward strike with your right sword arm.

(c) The push-off from the lunged position to the starting position must come from the foot. In water this whole action is slowed down, and there is time to do an optional straightening of the knee, whilst the foot is being returned to the starting position.

(d) Vary the angle so that you are lunging at 45 degrees, out to the right or left side.

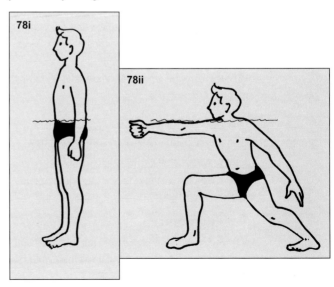

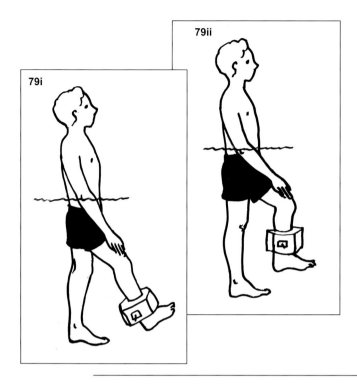

79. HAMSTRING PUMPS

Why do it?

To strengthen the hamstrings. It works the muscles concentrically when flexing, and eccentrically when straightening, providing a buoyant float is used.

Requirement

A 'weight', i.e. an inflated arm-band or ankle float.

Starting position

Lean with your back against the wall for support. Bring the right leg up to an angle of about 45 degrees, with a weight around the ankle. Place one or both hands on, or just above the knee, to ensure that the thigh remains stationary.

Movement

(a) Flex the right knee forcefully and quickly, so that it moves throughout the whole range of movement.

(b) Slowly allow the knee to return to the starting position.

80. HAMSTRING CURLS (BACKWARD KNEE BENDS)

Why do it? To work the muscles of the thighs – the hamstrings and the quadriceps.

Starting position

Stand with the feet and knees almost touching, and transfer the weight onto one leg.

Movement

(a) Bend the other knee up behind you, as though you are trying to kick your own bottom whilst keeping your knees still touching.

(b) Reverse the movement to return to the starting position.

Progression

1. Do it slowly and gently to warm up the knee.

2. Do it quickly to work the muscle harder.

3. Do it wearing a flipper to work the quadriceps and hamstrings harder.

Teaching point

If you wear a buoyant float round the foot or ankle, it becomes a different exercise. It will then work the quadriceps and not the hamstrings.

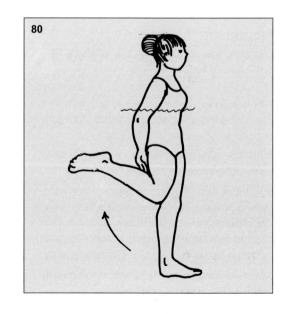

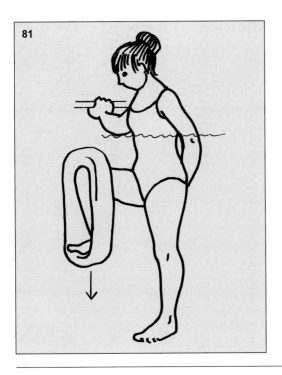

81. QUADS PUMP

Why do it?

This is powerful training for the quadriceps.

Requirement

A buoyant float, such as a woggle or a tyre.

Starting position

Stand with the feet together, and hold on to the side with one hand. Put the float under one foot.

Movement

(a) Allow the float to come up in the water as far as the knee will bend, trying to keep it as close to the trunk as possible.

(b) Without losing balance, push it down, leading with the heel, until you have returned to the starting position.

(c) Repeat, pushing down forcefully, but coming up slowly, until the thigh is tired.

82. RISES

Why do it? To strengthen the calf.

Requirement

For a full range ankle movement to strengthen the calf muscles, this exercise requires a step. It can be done starting off from the floor, but will not then use all the available range.

Starting position

Place the toes on the edge of a step, so that the heels are dangling out over space. Hold on with one hand.

Movement

(a) Rise up onto the toes of both feet, so that you are balanced at the edge of the step.

(b) Return to the starting position.

(c) If you are on a step, you can then lower your heels right down (whilst keeping the knees straight and the body balanced), so that the heels are now below the step.

Progression

Do it standing on one foot only. This is a really strong full-range calf exercise.

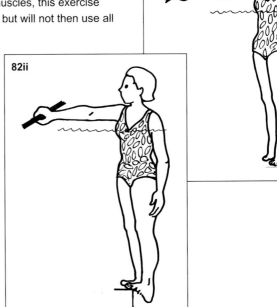

HIP AND/OR KNEE: ABDUCTION AND ADDUCTION

83. STRAIGHT LEG SWINGING

Why do it? To improve strength in the gluteal muscles, the hip adductor muscles and the quadriceps.

Starting position Hold on with one or both hands, with the feet together. Transfer all the weight onto the left leg.

Movement

(a) Keeping the tummy and the buttocks pulled in, lift the right leg out to the side. Make sure that the hip bone does not lift up, and that the leg is not coming forwards or backwards (83i).

(b) Return to the starting position.

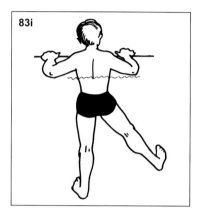
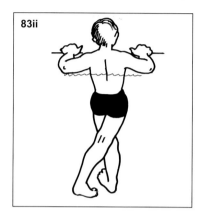

Progression

1.   Do it quicker to strengthen the muscles.

2.   Not to be done with a hip arthroplasty. Instead of returning the leg to the starting position, cross the left leg over in front of the right leg (83ii), possibly trying to touch the wall (you may need to stand nearer). Next time, cross the leg so that it goes behind the standing one. Continue so that in addition to parting, you are parting and crossing, alternately to the front and the rear of the standing leg. This movement opens up the facet joints of the lumbar spine. So, if there has been a back problem, this should be done with care.

84. SIDE LUNGES

Why do it?

If you happen to be a fencer, it may improve your performance! Otherwise, it works the hip abductor muscles with the knee flexors and extensors.

Starting position   Stand with the feet together and the weight on the left foot.

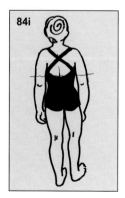
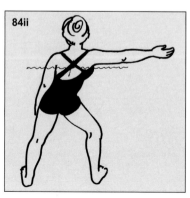

Movement

(a) Lunge out sideways, to the right, so that you take your right foot out to the side, and land on your right foot, and immediately bend the right knee. It is important that the feet remain parallel, and that the knee bends directly over the right foot (otherwise you may twist the knee).

(b) As you do this, reach out to the right side with your right hand.

(c) Push off with the right foot to spring back to the starting position.

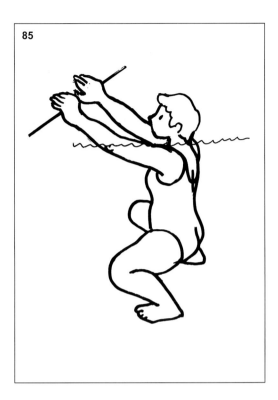

85

85. SQUATS

Why do it?

A truly primitive but pleasurable exercise – safe to do in water, but not on dry land!

Starting position

Stand in waist-high water, with the feet apart.

Movement

(a) Bend the knees so that the knees go over the feet, like a frog. You might find that you have to lift up the heels in order to bend the knees as low as is comfortable.

(b) Stand up to return to the starting position.

Progression

This exercise is important to Aquarobics. In order to facilitate remaining a bit longer in the squatting position, the arms can be given a movement to do, such as in 'Elbow circles' (page 164) or 'Pectoral arms' (page 166).

LEG ROTATION

86. LEG CIRCLES

Why do it?

It mobilizes the hip joint, and helps to warm up the region.

Starting position

Stand holding on to the side with the left hand. Stretch the right arm out to the side.

Movement

(a) Keeping your right knee straight, move that leg so as to draw an imaginary circle on the floor of the pool with the toes of your right foot.

(b) Increase the size of the circle, so as to allow your foot to lift up from the floor.

(c) After a few circles, reverse the direction of the movement.

(d) Turn round and repeat to the opposite side.

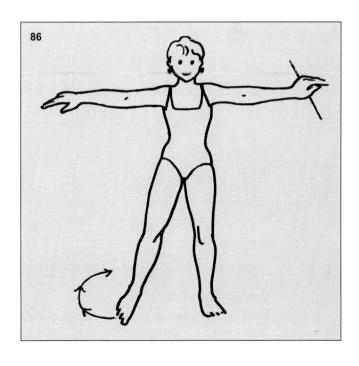

86

87. FIGURE-OF-EIGHT

Precaution

For those who have had a hip arthroplasty, this is only to be done under physiotherapy supervision, as some adduction over the midline is involved.

Why do it?

To tone up all the muscles of the hip and upper thigh.

Starting position

Hold on to the side of the pool with your right hand as though doing barre exercises.

Movement

Keeping your left leg straight, draw a figure-of-eight with your big toe, on the floor of the pool, making an anticlockwise circle in front of you and a clockwise circle behind you (87i).

Progression

1. Allow the knee to bend and the hip to twist, so that as you go forwards, the knee points inwards and vice versa (87ii). It is the size and speed of the movement which will determine whether this is primarily for muscle strength or joint flexibility.

2. It can be made even harder by placing an inflated arm-band, or ankle float around the ankle or foot.

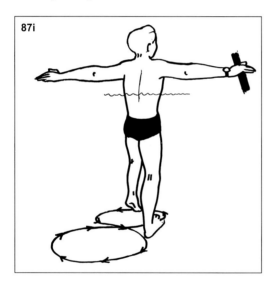

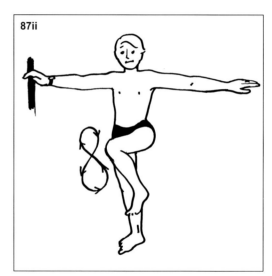

88. HIP PIVOTS

Precaution

This exercise should not be done by those who have had a hip arthroplasty.

Why do it?

To work the internal and external rotators of the hip joints.

Starting position

Stand close, and at right angles, to the side of the pool, holding on with your right hand. Bend up the left leg so that both hip and knee joints are at right angles. Place the left hand on the left hip bone.

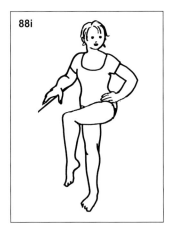

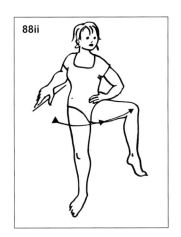

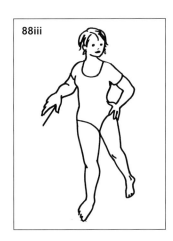

Movement

(a) Keeping the lower part of the leg vertical at all times, pivot the left leg round to try to get the left knee to touch the wall. The left hip bone should not move.

(b) When the leg is as far across the body as possible, reverse the direction of movement, so that the knee is brought outwards as far as possible (still keep the lower part of the leg vertical). The point of the knee should draw an arc of a circle of about 100 degrees (depending on how mobile the hip joint is).

Progression

Start as before, but when reversing the movement, stretch the left leg out diagonally behind you, so that it makes an angle of 45 degrees (an arabesque) (88iii). Again, the hip bone should not move, but there should be a smooth change from the stretched-out-behind position to the turned-in front-wall-touch position. This should not be done the first time, as this is a provocative exercise.

---

89. COSSACKSKI'S

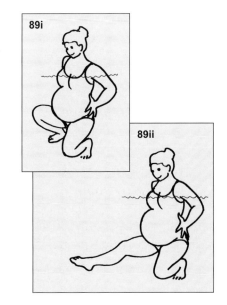

Why do it? This is a strong full-range quadriceps exercise, which is fun to do.

Precautions

Do not try this if you have meniscal problems, or locking knees. It must only be done in the water.

Starting position

Move into shallow water, preferably so that you are shoulder deep when you are in a full squat position. Bend both knees, keeping the spine vertical, so that you are squatting with both your knees pointing outwards.

Movement

(a) Transfer the weight onto one leg, and stand up on that leg. As you do this, kick out the other leg, like a Cossack.

(b) Change legs with each kick.

See also Helicopters (Exercise 34).

F LOCOMOTION EXERCISES

The following ten exercises involve different ways of moving around a pool. In individuals with no problems, they are useful as warm-up or aerobic exercises, depending on the speed they are done and the fitness levels of the people involved. They are also useful for the rehabilitation of normal locomotor function.

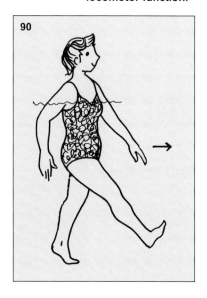

90. FORWARDS (HEEL–TOE) WALKING

Why do it?

This is the basic brick with which the other locomotor exercises are built. It is the way a small child first learns to walk – before their flexible, prehensile feet have been placed in rigid-soled shoes – causing the 'kipper feet' gait of most adults.

Movement

The stages of a complete forward step-cycle are:

(a) Only the heel hits the ground (with the front of the foot raised).

(b) As body weight moves forward, the foot is flat for an instant.

(c) The push-off comes from the ball of the big-toes. In the water, this upward push will cause the head to rise.

(d) As the leg goes forward, it is accompanied by the opposite arm.

The four stages should come together as a fluid, smooth movement, with the head bobbing up and down.

91. BACKWARDS (TOE–HEEL) WALKING

Why do it?

It is necessary to be able to move in all directions, and this involves walking backwards, sideways and all stages in between. Such movements improve coordination and balance.

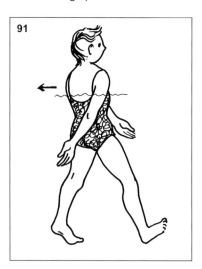

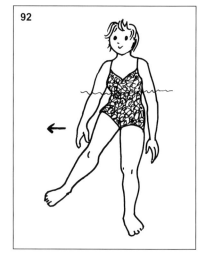

Movement

The stages of a complete backwards step-cycle are:

(a) The toes of one foot hit the ground.

(b) The rest of the foot follows.

(c) The opposite arm moves backwards in time with the leg.

92. WALKING SIDEWAYS

This is too obvious to explain in detail.

Keeping the trunk facing forwards, move sideways, by stepping out to the side, then bringing the feet together.

93. WALKING SIDEWAYS WITH LUNGES

When moving to the right (in waist-high water)

(a) Take a really wide stride. As you transfer your weight onto the right leg, flex the knee so that you are landing on a bent knee.

(b) At the same time reach out to the right with your right hand.

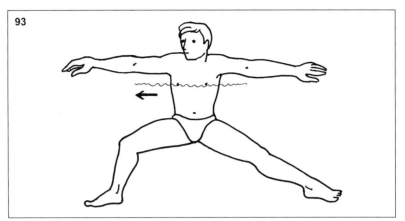

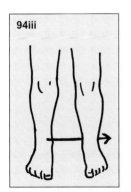

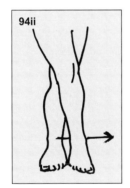

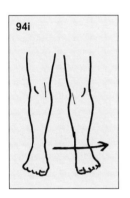

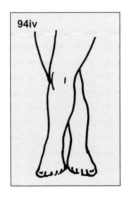

94. BRAIDING

This is a really useful exercise in rehabilitation, or when balance and coordination are poor.

Precaution

Not to be done by those who have had a hip arthroplasty, as it involves crossing the legs.

Movement

Progress sideways to the left across the pool facing one end at all times, keeping both feet facing forwards.

(a) Move the left leg out to the left (94i).

(b) Cross the right leg over in front of the ankle, so that the feet are touching each other – aligned like a pair of shoes placed with the right one on the left side, and vice versa (94ii).

(c) Step out again with the left leg to the left.

(d) This time, cross the right one behind the left one (94iv).

The whole manoeuvre follows a shape reminiscent of a grapevine.

95. SLOW MOTION RUNNING

This is rather pleasing to do, as (in the imagination at least), one is winning a gold-medal at the Olympics.

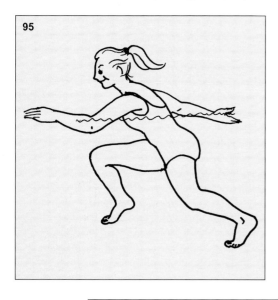

95

Movement

Mimic the action-replay of slow-motion running. The salient features are:

(a) This is a whole-body manoeuvre, as the trunk rotates to provide more force for the forward propulsion.

(b) The steps are much larger than when walking.

(c) There is a much greater movement in the knees and hips, which are brought right up.

(d) For some of the time, neither foot is on contact with the floor of the pool.

(e) The forward propulsion comes from the big toe.

(f) The trunk is kept straight, but tipped forward at an angle to the pool floor.

(g) The bent arms pump away in opposition to the legs, to assist in the rotation and propulsion.

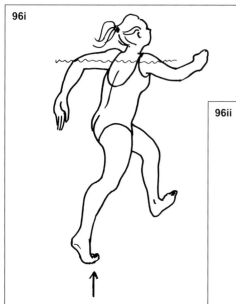

96i

96. SPRING RUNNING

Precaution

As this involves some jumping, it is important that the water is at least chest-high.

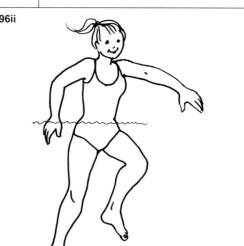

96ii

Movement

This is not a natural gait, but is designed to strengthen the calves and bring the bounce back into locomotion.

(a) The steps are kept small.

(b) The foot lands normally (the heel goes down first), but the push-off is exaggerated so that the body springs a little bit up and out of the water.

97. MARCHING

Movement

This exercise is exactly what it sounds like – an imitation of military marching, best done to military music.

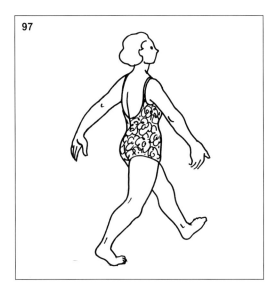

98. FLIPPER WALKING

This exercise is also what it sounds like. The client is told that they are wearing real (or imaginary) flippers. They will then have to walk forwards with a much exaggerated knee flexion – in order to prevent the edge of the flipper catching on the bottom of the pool and tripping them up.

This is useful in the re-education of those who have a stiff knee following surgery or immobilization. A real flipper is better (if it can be controlled without pain) but imaginary ones are also helpful in increasing the range of movement in the knee and ankle.

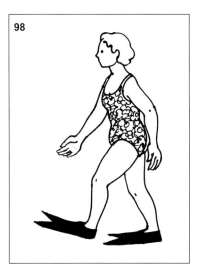

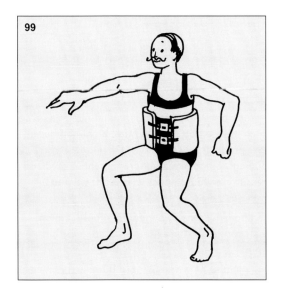

99. DEEP WATER RUNNING

Another descriptive title.

Precaution This is only for swimmers.

Requirement

It is theoretically possible for buoyant people to do this without equipment, but it is a skill that takes some practice to master. It is much easier to wear a buoyancy aid, such as a special belt designed for the purpose, or a wet-vest with built in buoyancy.

Why do it?

This is excellent cardiovascular work for fit people. There is no impact whatever, but a lot of whole-body muscle work.

Movement

Simply run in the deep end, either on the spot, or moving around, by alternating your arm and legs in exaggerated movement.

G BALANCE EXERCISES

Several of the exercises already listed are appropriate for use in balance re-training. Basically, any activity where balance is difficult, which is successfully undertaken without falling over, will help to re-train balance. For some people, merely standing in the pool in one spot, without holding on or being swept around by the turbulence, is sufficiently challenging. Other individuals can undertake complicated one-legged standing exercises, in which the centre of gravity is moved substantially (such as any of the leg swinging exercises), without losing balance.

Generally speaking, it is also harder to do exercises without holding on, especially if the movement has a large dimension. It is also harder to balance when the foot (or feet) is (are) kept still, than when they are permitted to 'hop' around. Many of the exercises already described have, or can be made to have, a balance component, simply by not holding on. Exercise 100 is an easy example.

100. ANKLE ROLLS

Why do it?

The following is a specific exercise which is aimed at balance training, as well as mobilizing the ankle.

Movement

Stand on one leg, with the other leg raised a little to the front. Circle the foot slowly round in the ankle, then reverse directions.

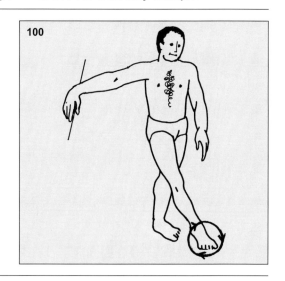

H AEROBIC COMBINATIONS

Chapters 2 and 13 explain why it is necessary to build up aerobic exercises and keep them at a peak. The following exercises are suggestions of ways in which this can be done. It must be remembered, though, that all muscular activity – in other words, all the preceding exercises – will increase the heart rate to some extent. These will probably be insufficient to achieve an improvement in cardiac function (aerobic capacity) in fit individuals, who will require the more specific exercises listed below.

Although it is impossible to quantify or standardise the effort that any one individual puts into any one exercise, an attempt has been made to grade them according to the effort required, (starting with the easiest).

In order to put load on the heart, both arms and legs will need to be working – but there is a choice of combinations of different movements. They have been arranged in a table as either arm or leg moves, starting with short lever (ie flexed knees and elbows) and progressing to long lever moves. Generally speaking, if the arms and legs are working together, it feels more comfortable to use the same length lever for both sets of limbs.

Table H.1 Aerobic combinations

	LEG MOVES		ARM MOVES	
	BASIC MOVE	**VARIATIONS**	**BASIC MOVE**	**VARIATIONS**
SHORT LEVER (Bent knees and elbows)	Running (either on the spot, or moving around with frequent directional changes)	Knees bent in front	Roly poly (circle the forearms round each other)	Reverse direction
		Feet towards the buttock, knees together	Jogging arms	Increase size of swing
		Knees to the sides	Push down arms with wrists dorsiflexed as paddles	The arms can move together or reciprocally
		Leap-frog knees	Leap-frog arms (both arms push down centrally)	Push down alternate arms

	LEG MOVES		ARM MOVES	
	BASIC MOVE	**VARIATIONS**	**BASIC MOVE**	**VARIATIONS**
SHORT LEVER (cont.)			Bicep–tricep curls	Rotating to alternate sides
LONG LEVER	Straight scissor kicks	Lean back	Straight elbows; scissor beating	
		Lean forwards	Try to touch opposite feet	
			Arm swinging; straight elbows	Either flexion and extension, or abduction and adduction

	LEG MOVES		ARM MOVES	
	BASIC MOVE	**VARIATIONS**	**BASIC MOVE**	**VARIATIONS**
LONG LEVER (cont.)			Punching the water	Speed it up, so as to make white water
	Side-swings (swing both straight legs to one side, then both to the other, head stays still)		Both arms swing to the same side as the legs, to maintain balance	
			Reaches – bend and stretch arms, singles or doubles	Out to sides, to the front or (hardest) to the ceiling
				Hands clap, to front or rear

	LEG MOVES		ARM MOVES	
	BASIC MOVE	**VARIATIONS**	**BASIC MOVE**	**VARIATIONS**
JUMPS	Tuck jumps	Keeping trunk vertical, bring knees up into sitting position and put down in the space of one jump	Clap hands under thighs	Both arms up over head, pull them both down into the water
	Frog jumps	Leap frog out of the water	Push down hard with both arms	
	Cross jumps	One knee up and across	Opposite elbow towards the knee	Take care not to jar knee and elbow together
	Twist jumps	Like the dance – twist your pelvis to one side as you jump	Twist your thorax and arms the other way	

LEG MOVES		ARM MOVES	
BASIC MOVE	**VARIATIONS**	**BASIC MOVE**	**VARIATIONS**

JUMPS (cont.)

LEG MOVES BASIC MOVE	VARIATIONS	ARM MOVES BASIC MOVE	VARIATIONS
		Pectoral arms	Elbows at right angles, forearms vertical. Bring into touch then horizontal abduction to part. Keep as much of arms as possible under water
Loops	Jump up high out of the water, rotating through 360 degrees before you land	Arms above the head, and use them to help you to turn	Those with long hair, take care!
Star jumps	Part the legs as you jump up. You may be able to get them together before you land. Be careful not to strain the adductor muscles	The arms start off down, and as you jump they go up and out as far as possible, to make the star shape	
Jump reaches	Both legs lift your body as high as possible out of the water	Both arms reach as high as possible above your head	

	LEG MOVES		ARM MOVES	
	BASIC MOVE	**VARIATIONS**	**BASIC MOVE**	**VARIATIONS**
WHOLE BODY MOVES	Skipping	Either moving around, or stationary with an imaginary rope	Swing the rope round	Be a child, skipping ropeless!
	Stride jumps and parts	Jump the legs apart and together. Cross the legs, alternating between in front and behind	The straight arms go out to the sides, then cross either in front or behind the body	
	Cross country skiing, on the spot, with a big stride	Mimic the motion – straight arms and legs glide as you alternate your limbs.	Keep the elbows and wrists still, and the fingers together. The hardest is to cut out the jump, and keep the head still.	The head will move up and down as you change position
	Head still: skiing	The same movement as the previous exercise	Make as much resistance as possible with the arms (hands as rigid paddles, elbows straight)	Do not allow your head to bob up and down
	The bell	One foot in front of the other. Jump from front to back foot, keeping trunk aligned	Both elbows and shoulders at right angles. Tip the trunk and arms forwards as you go forwards, then reverse	The whole movement vaguely resembles the shape of a bell

I FLEXIBILITY

MUSCLE STRETCHES

All stretches should be a slow gentle sustained stretch, lasting about 30 seconds to one minute. Please refer to the relevant section in Chapter 13.

101. CALF STRETCH

Structures stretched

The gastrocnemius muscle.

Starting position

Stand holding on to the pool with both hands, with one foot in front of the other, but both feet parallel to the way you are facing. Keeping the body vertical, the back knee straight and the back heel down, slowly bend the front knee. You should feel a stretch on the calf as you push against the wall. This is easier outside the water as you have more weight to push! Remember to do both legs!

Variation

Do it in pairs. It helps to get the extra weight, with the palms together, you can each push the other up and away, to increase the stretch.

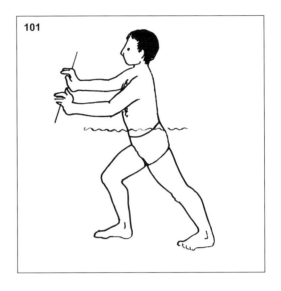

102. HAMSTRING STRETCH

Structures stretched

Hamstrings, sciatic nerve, shin muscles.

Starting position

Stand facing the pool wall and hold on with both hands to the sides with straight arms. Position your feet under your shoulders.

Movement

Place the toes of the right foot on the wall of the pool about 75–100 cm up from the floor, and lean forward a little. Get the stretch by straightening your right knee, and trying to get your right heel against the wall. If you cannot feel a stretch down the back of your leg, then raise the foot. Keep your back straight, and stick out your buttock.

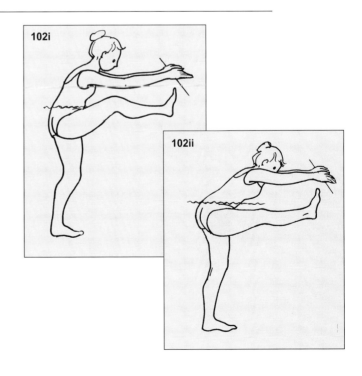

103. QUADRICEPS STRETCH

Structures stretched

The quadriceps muscles, especially rectus femoris.

Starting position

Stand on one leg, holding the other foot around the ankle with the hand on that side, so that the leg is held behind you.

Movement

While keeping the body upright, slowly pull that leg farther back. You will feel a pull on the muscles at the front of the thigh. Make sure that the knees remain close to each other and keep the lumbar spine tucked flat.

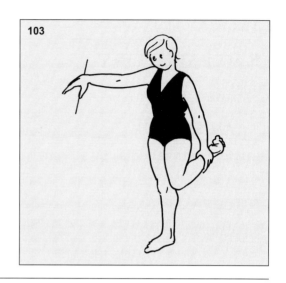

103

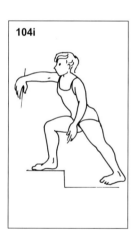

104i

104ii

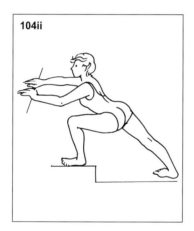

104iii

104. PSOAS STRETCH

Structures stretched　The psoas muscle.

Starting position

This can only be done in the water if there is a step or a suitable rung of a ladder on which to put your foot or, if it is done in pairs (104iii). Otherwise do it on dry land.

Individually

Put the right foot on a step about 35 cm high, with the knee bent, and put the other leg as far behind you as possible.

Movement

Bend your body forwards, but keeping the upper body vertical. Slowly stretch, and you will feel the pull in the groin.

In pairs

Get into shallow water, and face each other. The helper interlocks her fingers, which act as a foot support. The other person places one foot in the palms of the helper, and both hands on their shoulders. The other leg should be as far behind as possible.

Movement

They then bend their front knee, to get into the position illustrated.

General Slow Static Stretches

105. BACK REACHING

Structures stretched

Shoulder joints and triceps muscle.

Starting position

Stand with the feet apart for stability.

Movement

Try and get your fingers to touch behind your back, one going from the top and the other one from the bottom, as illustrated.

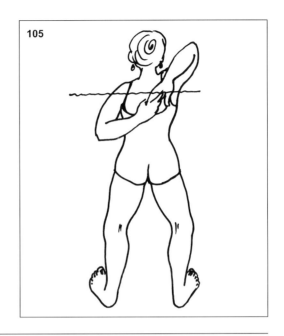

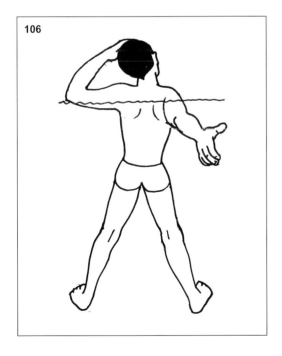

106. ARM AND CERVICAL NERVE STRETCH

Structures stretched

Lower cervical nerves, shoulder muscles and joint, neck and arm muscles, wrist.

Starting position

Put your hand against the pool wall so that the wrist is as far back as possible, and the fingers straight. The elbow should be straight and the entire arm turned outwards away from the body. The arm should be behind the trunk, and the shoulder not hunched up. The neck should then be bent to the side away from the arm. You should be aware of a stretching feeling in the arm and sometimes down to the hand. Be careful!

107. ARM AND SPINE STRETCH

Structures stretched

Shoulder, elbow, wrist and finger joints, and the upper spine.

Starting position

Stand and clasp your hands in front of you, close to your chest.

Movement

Slowly raise both hands as high as you can above your head. At the same time try and make yourself taller, ie, push the top of your head up, but keep your chin tucked in. Hold the stretch for a few seconds, and then release it, and turn your interlocked hands so that the palms are upwards. Now wind the stretch on again (if you can), and you will feel even more pull all the way down to the middle of your back. Your arms should be behind your ears!

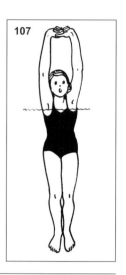

DYNAMIC STRETCHES

108. QUADRICEPS FLIP

Structures stretched

The quadriceps and buttock muscles, the hip joints, the whole spine.

Starting position

Stand in water about midriff depth. Hold on with your right hand.

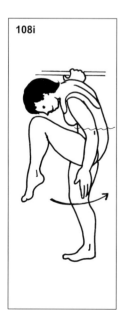

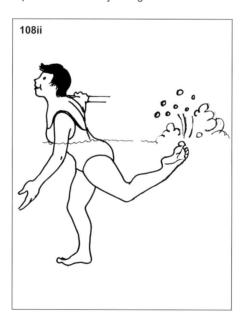

Movement

(a) Bring your left knee up in front of you, so that the higher it is, the more it is bent. Bring your head down as though to try to touch your knee with your forehead (108i). (DO NOT PUSH THROUGH PAIN!)

(b) Now straighten yourself up and move the straight left leg downwards and backwards until it is as far behind you as possible. Allow your upper body to tip forward somewhat, and arch your spine, but keep your chin tucked in.

(c) When your leg is as far back as it wants to go, then finish off by quickly bending your knee with a pointed foot (108ii). This dynamic 'flick' should cause some water to lift up into the air to make a splash!

109. PIKE SQUATS AND STRETCHES

Structures stretched

Hamstrings, lower back, hips, sciatic nerve and shoulder joints.

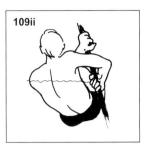

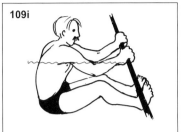

Starting position

You can only do this exercise if you can hold onto the edge of the pool, and the pool wall is vertical. Hold on to the side of the pool, (or a rail), with your hands shoulder-width apart. Your hands should not move throughout the exercise. Place both feet as high as you can against the pool wall (109i).

Movement

(a) At certain points of this exercise you should try to get into the pike position with your heels against the wall and your knees straight. If you cannot achieve this then lower both feet a little bit.

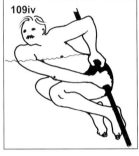

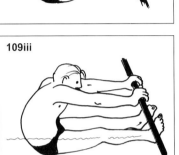

(b) Bend both knees and pull your body to the right, so that the right cheek of your buttock touches the pool wall close to your right hand (109ii). You should be almost sitting on your feet.

(c) Immediately change direction, so as to return to the starting position, but pause for a couple of seconds as you go through the central 'pike' (109iii).

(d) Continue to move to the left, and carry on as before.

This exercise is one of almost continuous smooth slow motion. The only exception is the pause as you 'wind up' the pike stretch!

110. UNCURL AND BOW STRETCH

This is a good exercise with which to end a session. It is a re-mobilizer after a relaxation.

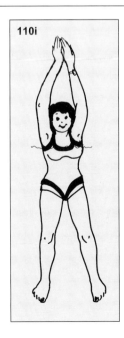

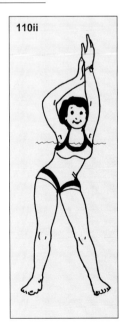

Structures stretched

The spine, ribs and shoulders.

Starting position

Stand in waist- to chest-high water, with the feet shoulder-width apart. Stretch both arms above the head, with the palms touching.

Movement

(a) Slide up the left palm, and pull down the right one, as though pulling down a bow string.

(b) As you do this, allow the hips to move to the right, so that the whole body, but especially the chest and pelvis, is in a sideways curve.

(c) Return to the midline and slowly stretch the other way.

J PELVIC FLOOR CONTRACTIONS

This may seem an illogical place to put Pelvic Floor Contractions (Exercise 111), but no place seems ideal. These exercises fit quite well into the relaxation, cool-down period of a session, so they have been placed here at the end of the Exercise section, which coincides with the end of the Aquarobic work-out. The fact that they do not fit conveniently anywhere else must not detract from the importance of good control of these muscles in the maintenance of healthy physiological functioning.

Possibly because one is teaching how to contract the muscles of the pelvic floor in an aquatic environment, at the end of a class, by which time you (it is hoped) have the respect and confidence of the clients, and have at least shared one good laugh during the session, this task is easier and does not seem to infringe so much into personal privacy. Visualization is a useful teaching method.

III. PELVIC FLOOR CONTRACTIONS

Pelvic Floor

Returning the stretched and damaged pelvic floor to its pre-natal function is probably the most important aspect to post-natal exercise. It is important that this is correctly taught. It is helpful to explain the anatomy, as many women are ignorant about their internal organs.

The following explanation has been adapted from the Kingston Incontinence Support Group.

The pelvic floor is a dynamic structure made up of layers of muscles which interweave and stretch like a hammock from the tail bone, between our legs to the pubic bones at the front. The function is two-fold, firstly to support the uterus, bladder and bowel and secondly to prevent leakage from the latter two, especially when coughing or lifting. When the pelvic floor muscles are contracted, they work with the urethral and anal sphincter muscles to close the canals, acting as a tap. When you relax the muscles, the tap opens and the bladder muscle (detrusor) contracts to expel urine, or the abdominal muscles contract to initiate a bowel movement.

The best way to learn to do pelvic floor exercises is by using your index and middle finger and inserting it into your vagina, whilst in the bath or propped up in bed. Gently tighten the muscles until you can feel the vagina tighten around your fingers. If the muscle is weak there will only be a flicker, but if it is stronger, you will feel a definite bulging.

Try to avoid squeezing your legs and buttocks together.

Find out how many seconds you can hold the contraction, and how often you can repeat it. The muscles tire very quickly, so a 4 second rest between contractions is necessary.

This is the starting point for your exercise programme. You do not need to use your fingers once you are sure that the muscles are working properly. You can exercise in any position, and at all times of the day. However, if the muscle is very weak it is easiest to exercise lying down, and in the mornings.

The aim of the exercise is to be stronger for longer and faster! Tighten the muscles before coughing, sneezing or lifting.

An alternative imagery is to imagine having diarrhoea whilst on the M1, 5 miles short of the next service station. Squeeze the back passage as though trying to hold on (making sure not to tighten the other unwanted muscle groups). Next bring the contraction slightly forward, as though trying to stop the flow of urine.

The best way to check whether you are being effective is by using natural biofeedback – either by using a finger and feeling the squeeze – or during intercourse when the partner can confirm whether or not there is a muscle contraction. These testing methods are by verbal instructions only and are not intended to be carried out in the pool during an aquatic exercise session!

When the pelvic floor contraction is mastered, it should be practised so as to work both the aerobic and the power fibres of the pelvic floor muscles. To work the former, tighten and hold the contraction for 4 seconds. Repeat until the muscles are tired – try and get up to 10 seconds hold if you can, repeated eight to ten times. To work the power fibres, go for a maximum contraction, but only hold it for a second. Repeat only four or five times. Breathing should be normal throughout.

Instructions

Imagine you are in a car on the M25, and you are suddenly aware not only that you have diarrhoea, but that you wish to urinate. You know that it is at least 10 miles to the next Service Station!

You will automatically tighten up the muscles of the pelvic floor – that is the sling of muscles around the back passage and the vagina (or, if it is a mixed class, and the muscles that control the passing of urine). These muscles are very important, and they need to be exercised just like all the other muscles in the body. If they get weak, you can leak urine when you cough or laugh.

You might say: 'So let us all try and do this now. I want to you to pull in these muscles and hold them in for five seconds. There are three ways to check whether you are doing this properly. Next time you pass water, see if you can stop the flow. It is not a good idea to do this too often, but it is useful as an occasional check that you have the correct control. Secondly, insert one or two fingers into your vagina, and see if you can feel a slight squeeze. Thirdly, if you have a partner, you can get feedback during sex. It is said that making these muscles stronger should help your sex life!'

K RELAXATION

Providing that there is no danger of clients getting cold, floating with buoyancy aids is a perfect way to relax and finish a class. Those people with a high body fat content will probably be able to lie back and float without assistance, but most people will require the help of buoyancy aids such as woggles, floats or belts, or manual assistance to maintain the supine position in unsalted water.

112. RELAXATION IN PAIRS

This either requires close handling, or buoyancy aides. The former is not always culturally acceptable, and may be embarrassing, especially if it is a non-medical class for both men and women.

Method 1. Without buoyancy aids

Person A is asked to lie down on their back, whilst person B ducks down into the water, so that it is at their shoulder level. They then assist by standing on A's left side, and preparing to place their right hand under the back of A's head. At the same time, B places their left hand just below the small of the back, which is on the centre of buoyancy. B then tells A to relax their legs, so that they bend a little, and flop outwards. They then tell them to relax completely all over (having first checked whether they mind putting their ears and hair in the water) and while supporting them, move them randomly and gently around the surface of the pool, taking care not to crash into another couple or the sides. (It is a little like horizontal ballroom dancing!)

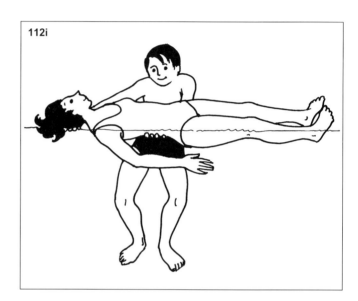

112i

Method 2. Using a woggle or two, or other appropriate aid.

Person A lies down and Person B slips the aid under them. If they only have one, it needs to be in the small of the back, but if two are available, it is better to place one as a head support under the neck, and the other one under the knees (112ii). B then moves the floating, relaxed A around the pool, as above.

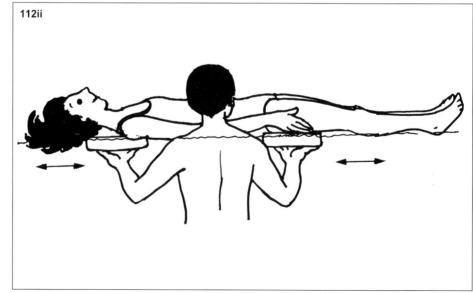

112ii

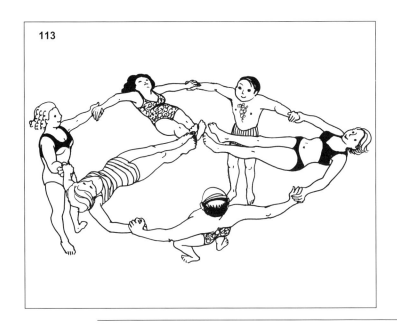

113

113. RELAXATION IN A CIRCLE

Requirement

A group of at least six people.

Movement

The group is told to get into a circle, hold hands and move around sideways so that the circle is rotating at a comfortable speed. Every second person is then told to lie down, with their feet towards the centre of the circle. The momentum of the moving circle will keep the people horizontal, although their feet will swing over to one side. They are told to relax completely and be pulled along by their vertical colleagues. Do not change the direction of movement while people are floating.

114. RELAXATION IN A LINE

This involves a lot of handling by clients of each other, and may therefore not be appropriate in a group of younger people, who are often less orientated to touching than older people. It may be inappropriate in some mixed sex groups.

Movement

Everybody stands in a line, a little way apart and facing the same way, with their shoulders in the water to prevent any back strain. The person at the head of the line lies down on his/her back and floats with the assistance of the second person, who places one hand under the head, and the other hand in the small of the back. They are then passed from person to person down the line, and when they reach the end, they are gently helped to stand up. As soon as the person has been passed along the line through the first three or four people, the next person can follow them.

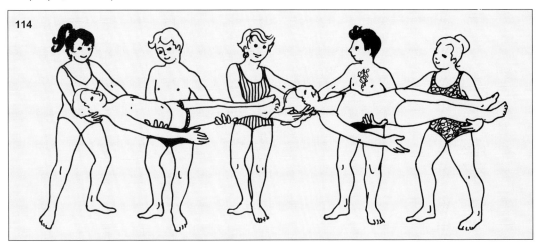

114

Index

Numbers in italic refer to tables or illustrations. Named exercises can be found under 'exercises'.